The
Psych 101 Series

Series

James C. Kaufman, PhD, Series Editor
Neag School of Education
University of Connecticut

Linda Gomberg, JD, PhD is an associate professor of forensic psychology at The Chicago School of Professional Psychology in Irvine and Los Angeles, California. She is an active member of the State Bar of California and earned her doctorate in psychology with an emphasis in media psychology at the Fielding Graduate University. She has practiced transactional law and continues to consult on contractual issues. Dr. Gomberg taught legal writing, contracts, agency and partnership, remedies, and civil procedure at the law school level and created the first academic support program for her law school students. She has also taught English in the public schools and media ethics for graduate students. She has presented on social media in the courts for Division 46 of the American Psychological Association and as continuing education for Licensed Masters in Family Therapy (MFT), and on sex offenders for senior undergraduate students from CETYS University in Northern Mexico (with Dr. Adam Yerke); she has also presented on and written about domestic violence. Dr. Gomberg coauthored (with Dr. Carolyn Sachs) a chapter on intimate partner sexual abuse in *Intimate Partner Violence: A Bio-Psycho-Social Approach*. She has also published in *Orange County Lawyer* and *Western State University Law Review*. She is currently the Southern California Chair of The Chicago School Institutional Review Board, a member and past Chair of the Ethics Committee of Division 46 (Media Psychology and Technology) and a member of Division 41 (American Psychology-Law Society) of the American Psychological Association. She serves as Chair of The Chicago School of Professional Psychology's California Institutional Review Board, and is a member of several other school and department committees.

Forensic Psychology 101

Linda Gomberg, JD, PhD

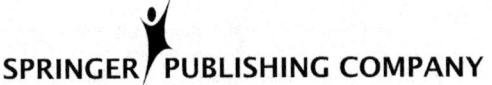

SPRINGER PUBLISHING COMPANY

Springer Publishing Company, LLC
11 West 42nd Street
New York, NY 10036
www.springerpub.com

Acquisitions Editor: Kate Dimock
Compositor: diacriTech

ISBN: 978-0-8261-4074-6
ebook ISBN: 978-0-8261-4075-3

18 19 20 / 5 4 3 2

The author and the publisher of this Work have made every effort to use sources believed to be reliable to provide information that is accurate and compatible with the standards generally accepted at the time of publication. The author and publisher shall not be liable for any special, consequential, or exemplary damages resulting, in whole or in part, from the readers' use of, or reliance on, the information contained in this book. The publisher has no responsibility for the persistence or accuracy of URLs for external or third-party Internet websites referred to in this publication and does not guarantee that any content on such websites is, or will remain, accurate or appropriate.

Library of Congress Cataloging-in-Publication Data
Names: Gomberg, Linda, author.
Title: Forensic psychology 101 / Linda Gomberg.
Description: New York, NY: Springer Publishing Company, LLC, [2018] |
    Includes bibliographical references.
Identifiers: LCCN 2018000372| ISBN 9780826140746 | ISBN 9780826140753 (e-book)
Subjects: | MESH: Forensic Psychiatry | United States
Classification: LCC RA1151 | NLM W 740 | DDC 614/.15—dc23 LC record available at
https://lccn.loc.gov/2018000372

Contact us to receive discount rates on bulk purchases.
We can also customize our books to meet your needs.
For more information please contact: sales@springerpub.com

Printed in the United States of America.

This book is dedicated to my family: My husband, children, grandchildren, and the babies. I am blessed that there are too many of you to name, but you are what it's all about and . . .
I love you more . . .

Many months pass between the submission of a manuscript and its publication.
During this time our oldest daughter lost her brave fight with cancer. This book, then, is also dedicated to the memory of our amazing and beautiful Dorinne.

Contents

CONTENTS

Foreword

Recently, I met with the president of a college where I was trying to establish a collaborative partnership. I always begin my instruction with an explanation of the locations of our campuses primarily because our flagship campus is located in Chicago; however, we have campuses in other locations such as those in Southern California, where we are. I then proceed to discuss the various programs and the types of degrees offered. I elaborated on the various direct and nondirect services our graduate psychology programs could offer, and the president was genuinely engaged. I talked about our Clinical Forensic Psychology program, the faculty in our department, the curriculum, and other academic and logistical aspects. I should add that this president's undergraduate degree concentration was psychology, and while her PhD emphasis was student development, her master's degree had a dual focus on counseling and student development; given her background, I knew she was familiar with the clinical and nonclinical aspects of the field of psychology. Although I knew she had an understanding of the field and that my explanation of our program offerings held her attention, I anticipated the question that is always asked, and then it came: *What exactly is forensic psychology?*

I recall my first encounter with Linda at a MMPI-2 training intensive during our graduate studies. Based on our outward appearances, most would probably wonder why we gravitated to each other. We are different in many ways with regard to basic demographics such as race, ethnicity, and age, probably the most notable statistic:

Linda takes great pleasure in reminding me that she is old enough to be my mother, and at times has acted as such. However, I believe that what transcends those differences is our mutual curiosity about how systems and theories are driven by our analytical approach. We are also rarely satisfied with the short answers about why things are the way they are, mostly because we believe in the Socratic philosophy of questioning. We are not easily impressed by *experts*, having seen our fair share of people calling themselves that or being designated as such, only to learn the irreparable damage those *experts* have caused. We are highly critical—but if you pass our litmus tests, then we will fully support the theory, idea, or position. As we engaged our facilitator and our colleagues during the training, I came to admire and appreciate Linda's contribution to the discussion from the *lawyer's* perspective, and I would like to think that she appreciated my perspective as well. I knew then that we would have many more conversations about the law and psychology. What I had not expected was how I began widening my viewpoint of psychology to include a more substantive understanding of pertinent legal aspects. In fact, at the time I had not realized that much of what I was doing for myself as a mental health professional, for my clients while acting at times as their advocate, and for the profession of psychology was firmly rooted in and shaped by the law. One of the benefits of having Linda in my life was getting the legal perspective and knowledge without having to attend law school.

My graduate studies focused on clinical psychology; however, I worked with a number of forensic populations before, during, and after my doctoral program. Due to my experiences in forensic settings, I believe that all clinicians would benefit from knowing about what forensic psychology is. In fact, while forensic psychology is not a new area of focus, with the *Specialty Guidelines for Forensic Psychology* having been developed and published by the American Psychological Association (APA) in 1991, the APA recognized it as an official specialty only in 2001, with subsequent recertification occurring in 2008. One of the primary challenges with the guidelines is that the goals set forth are "aspirational" and, therefore, differ from standards, which are mandatory. With this in mind, there is probably great variability in the depth and breadth of training and practical application of forensic psychology. I have great confidence in our profession and am equally confident that excellent resources are readily available, because I have attended trainings and own forensic resources. Nevertheless, I have yet to find a singular forensic resource created by a lawyer with a psychologically informed perspective. *Forensic Psychology 101* is a resource that is essential reading for those new to the area as well as for seasoned professionals.

I know that one of Linda's dreams was to write a book, and I was thrilled when she told me the circumstances that led to her dream becoming a reality. I believe that Linda's scholarly contribution to the field will be a great benefit. When Linda approached me about contributing to her book, I was honored and eagerly accepted. It is my hope that as you read this book, your knowledge of forensic psychology will increase and that you will appreciate the intersection of law and psychology as much as I have come to appreciate the intersection of the lawyer and the psychologist who formed an unlikely friendship, which remains to this day.

Loren M. Hill, PhD
Department Chair
Director of the Forensic Training Institute
Clinical Forensic Psychology Department
The Chicago School of Professional Psychology
Southern California

Preface

THE GOAL AND THE AUDIENCE

Forensic Psychology 101 is for students who want to know more about the law, students who want to know more about a psychology sub-specialty, and anyone who just wants to know more. The goal is to take the reader on his or her own learning experience, to create an environment of inquiry. The goal is not to answer questions; it is to create them.

When I first began writing this book, I intended for it to be an overview (after all, it is 101) of the topic at hand: forensic psychology. It was to be the book I wished my master's- and doctoral-level students had read prior to enrolling in a forensic psychology graduate program, the book that would provide a firm foundation on which they could build their knowledge during the years to come. It could also be the book I handed to friends and acquaintances who asked me to explain forensic psychology to them.

THE BACKGROUND

I expected to cover the breadth of the topic with little or no depth—that would and could come later for those who actually did enroll in a graduate program. For those who just wanted to learn what forensic psychology was all about, this book would be enough, or maybe it would whet their appetite to learn more. Initially, I made the mistake of doing what I cautioned first my law students and later my forensic psychology students never to do: I assumed, presumed, and predicted. I assumed I could glide through the chapters addressing the major topics in forensic psychology and plug in the references as required. After all, I write and teach my school's introductory course. I presumed I knew everything there was to know about the major topics that would be covered. I have books filled with notes and PowerPoint presentations that I created for my students as well as other presentations on social media, social psychology, and sex offenders. Finally, I predicted the writing would be easy. I enjoy writing, taught English, and actually have a master's degree in the subject.

But as I began the process and found myself checking and rechecking laws, cases, and the current state of psychological theory on almost every topic I decided to write about, I became so engrossed in what I was learning that the actual writing had to wait while the notes piled up. State laws changed in January; the United States (U.S.) Supreme Court handed down decisions in June. Many of us continued to wait for a new *Diagnostic and Statistical Manual of Mental Disorders (DSM)* to be published. From the time *DSM-5* was published in 2013, "everyone" was sure the fifth version would soon be replaced by a 5.1. Of course, we are still waiting. I was accumulating a great amount of information and soon realized that the topic of forensic psychology is so broad and deep that there would always be something else to learn.

One of the first things I learned is that titles matter. In some states, including mine, calling oneself a psychologist when unlicensed is misleading and prohibited. Therefore, unlike some of the psychologists I interviewed, I cannot call myself a forensic psychologist—at least in my state. Although I am licensed to practice law and have a PhD in psychology that makes me license eligible, I have never logged the requirements to sit for the exam.

The next thing I learned, however, is that there are many ways to "practice" forensic psychology, and I have a dream job that allows me to do just that. I am a teacher of forensic psychology who is constantly fascinated by and learning more about the intersection of law and psychology and wondering how we were ever able to distinguish the two. I am a researcher who, with my students, is constantly finding new constructs that lend themselves to law and psychology. Although I started by studying privacy through the lenses of psychology and the law, together my students and I have researched the legal and psychological aspects of empathy, false confessions, confidence, child custody, and all forms of deception detection in various contexts and through the perspectives of law enforcement, juries, witnesses, and the lay public. The possibilities are endless, and forensic psychology students are curious and creative.

So what this book became is my learning experience. There are no limits to the possibilities of subtopics in forensic psychology, and studying one topic gives rise to wanting to know more about a topic raised within that interest area—and so on. There are questions everywhere, and the answers invariably raise more questions, and that is what forensic psychology is really about.

CONTENT

The book is divided into three parts. Part I gives an overview and describes the origins of forensic psychology. Chapter 1 is a history lesson of sorts in that the roots of psychology and the law are explored individually and in their coming together. One of the more well-known cases, *The Queen v. McNaughton* (1843), set the scene for the origins of forensic psychology some time before psychologists started thinking about the value of psychology in the courts. In reality, it is one of the few times that the law was actually ahead of psychology. Chapter 2 builds on this foundation by examining the origins of our legal system, the United States Constitution and the ways that its provisions have been utilized by the three branches of government, particularly by the courts. Beginning with Chapter 3, the last chapter in Part I, the chapters each describe one aspect of forensic psychology. Chapter 3 brings the first two chapters together by describing how two major constructs, context and perception, are integral to understanding both disciplines.

The four chapters of Part II specifically address the role of forensic psychology in the courts by beginning with the topics that seem to be of the utmost interest to readers and students: criminal matters and ethical issues. Chapter 4 includes various types of crimes, pleas, and punishment relevant to forensic psychology issues and practice. Many of these types of cases eventually get to the U.S. Supreme Court and provide not only endless publicity for the parties and attorneys, but also opportunities for forensic psychologists who participate in the courts in these criminal matters in various capacities. Chapter 5 parallels the information given in Chapter 4 with a discussion of civil matters, including the roles of witness testimony (both expert and eye) and jury selection. A nationally recognized expert is profiled in Chapter 5. Forensic psychologists' roles in family court are varied and are the subject of Chapter 6. Such topics as "psychological autopsies," suicide prevention, and the forensic psychologist's role in the complex matters presented by our changing society and family systems are also addressed. Part II concludes with Chapter 7 and the forensic psychologist's role in the juvenile justice system. Although there are always some overlaps and some omissions, each of the chapters in Part II identifies specific roles for the forensic psychologist within the legal context of the chapter and conjectures about what that role might have been in each of the illustrative cases.

Finally, Part III clarifies and expands on the roles of the forensic psychologist and attorney in court proceedings. Chapter 8 provides an outline of the similarities and differences between the professions, and also distinguishes the role of the clinical or therapist psychologist. Chapter 9, as the final chapter in this book, appropriately addresses the growing future of forensic psychology. Areas that are not necessarily court based, but are certainly areas of interest and work for the forensic psychologist, are introduced. The final chapter completes the circle that was the objective of this book: By the time it is read, there should be little doubt as to what forensic psychology is and which roles the forensic psychologist can have that distinguish her or him from all other mental health professionals.

Each chapter begins with an overview and an explanation of how forensic psychology is a function of that topic. An important part of each chapter is the relevant case or sometimes cases that explain the chapter topics. The cases are presented as "briefs" so that the important facts, issues, and holdings are readily noted.

The most effective method of explaining how forensic psychology works would be to hear about it from a forensic psychologist.

The "Focus on Careers" sections begin with Chapter 3 and continue through Chapter 7. At least one forensic psychologist actively working in that particular area is profiled in each of the chapters. Chapter 8 changes the perspective, however, and introduces two working attorneys whose practices have always included the input of forensic psychologists.

Beginning with Chapter 2 and continuing throughout each chapter, an "In the News" section is featured. Newspapers, technological media, and other news sources are filled with examples of the need for forensic psychology and forensic psychologists. The chapters all conclude with a Summary and Discussion Questions. They are questions that have no right or wrong answers—questions I would love to hear responses to, questions I wish I could discuss.

So, please join me in learning the basics, meeting the professionals, and entering the world of a very special profession. You will find there is something for everyone, and always something more to explore!

Acknowledgments

irst and foremost, I want to acknowledge the only person who read every single chapter of this book as I wrote and rewrote it. While he certainly bears no responsibility for whatever may not work in these pages, he deserves accolades for patience in reading, suggesting, and honesty. So, to my husband, Raymond Gomberg, MD: Thank you!

This book would never have been written if not for Jerri Lynn Hogg, PhD, and Loren M. Hill, PhD. Jerri Lynn has been a one-person cheering section, encouraging my writing and professional activities since we were students, when she became my professor, and as colleagues who are a very close 3,000 miles apart. If not for her, I would not have met Debra Riegert of Springer, who deserves not only acknowledgment, but also a major thank you for her encouragement, enthusiasm, and focus on what this book should be. Was it luck that Jerri Lynn and I happened to "stop by" at the Springer table after presenting at APA in Denver in 2016? If so, I am happy to acknowledge my very good fortune in having the right friend and colleague and the right editor.

It is similar to the good fortune I experienced when I met Loren Hill during my first year of graduate school. She was transitioning from law enforcement to psychology to teaching, and I was transitioning from teaching and law practice to psychology. How many years later was it when Loren said: Have I got a job for you! If not for Loren Hill, I would not have my dream job teaching in a Forensic Psychology Graduate program for The Chicago School of Professional Psychology. She was and is my friend, my colleague, and now the chair of my department. If my dream job had not materialized, this book certainly would never have been written.

If not for Loren Hill, I also would not have known several of the busy professionals who were kind enough to be interviewed for this book. I am honored to call Drs. Jim Earnest, Jay Finkelman, Clive Kennedy, Sammie Williams, and Adam Yerke my colleagues. They are all experts, and their stories could each fill a book. Dr. Trisha Elloyan and Michael Fisher were both my students, many years apart and in two different professional schools. Trisha was my student in the Clinical Forensic PsyD program at The Chicago School of Professional Psychology, and Michael preceded her by more than two decades when he was my law student at Western State University College of Law. I have learned so much from both of them. I have also learned a lot from the other attorney whom I interviewed for this book: Stephan DeSales not only fascinates with his stories of his varied criminal cases, he also provided me with an idea for a whole section of this book, leading me to look into cases and psycholegal defenses I may not have thought of without the suggestion. Finally, thank you to Stuart Hochwert for time and expertise in guiding me through the initial process. How fortunate I am that my children have such accomplished friends.

To all of those people and to my students past, present, and future, you are my idea people, and I am most appreciative.

1

An Overview of Forensic Psychology: The Origins

The History of Forensic Psychology

OVERVIEW

Whether we make our living in clinical practice, academia, research, or a combination of these fields, as psychology professionals we tend to label, sort, categorize, and define. For clinicians, this may be the best path to take to arrive at a diagnosis and/or course of treatment, which usually requires matching symptoms to criteria listed in the latest edition of the *Diagnostic and Statistical Manual of Mental Disorders* (*DSM*) of the American Psychiatric Association, the "bible" universally used by mental health clinicians regardless of theoretical orientation, degree level, or theoretical approach. For the practitioner, the *DSM* has already provided the sorting and categorizing. For academics, who search for how best to explain a construct to students, while being mindful of what has worked in the past and what needs updating and revision for today's students, the sorting, labeling, and awareness of changing definitions are ever-present concerns. For pure researchers, the task might be the testing process through which a new **probability** is created; researchers need to establish parameters by explaining their methods, operationalizing terminology, and finally sorting and categorizing their findings (Popper, 2002). Rarely, however, in discussions about psychology (or within courses with "psychology" in their titles) is the discipline mentioned without a preceding adjective. To name just a very few examples, those modifiers provide us with social psychology, cognitive psychology, experimental psychology, developmental psychology, abnormal psychology, media psychology, and even general psychology (American Psychological Association [APA], n.d.). The APA encourages this labeling and categorizing by dividing itself into 54 individually named divisions. Although members can and do belong to more than one division, their choices most often are determined by their interests, experience, and education. In fact, speaking just for myself, I belong to Divisions 41 and 46 of the APA. I belong to the former, officially named the **American Psychology-Law Society**, for several reasons: I teach in a graduate-level forensic psychology program; I am an attorney with a juris doctor degree and have a PhD in psychology, and my professional, academic, and research interests all seem to have a connection to the nexus of psychology and the law. I joined and am active in Division 46, the Society for Media Psychology and Technology, because my PhD in psychology was earned with an emphasis in media. Further, the dual memberships speak to my overlapping professional/academic interests. This area is forensic psychology—a subset of social psychology that combines the understanding of law and the study of human behavior. In my case, forensic psychology was the natural evolution of my professional interests. Whatever your reasons, I hope you find your place in the profession as well.

Of course, we all know labels are not all that unusual in any profession. Medical doctors divide their interests into specialties; lawyers specialize and join bar association divisions that best describe their area of civil or criminal practice; school teachers are equipped to teach certain grades and/or subjects. For these and other professions, however, the specialty is often self-explanatory and evident in their one-word titles: Pediatricians treat children, cardiologists treat hearts, neurologists treat brains and spinal cords, and so forth. Does anyone need an explanation when told she is talking to a criminal defense attorney or a family law attorney? These professions and their specialties are self-defining.

This is not the case when first meeting a psychologist.[1] An individual who introduces himself as a social psychologist, for example, may be a person who has completed a program with an emphasis in social psychology teaching in a media psychology program. It is the interaction and/or influence of media on behavior that leads to this classification (APA, n.d.; Ferguson, 2016). Even then, two types of media psychologists are recognized; in fact, media psychology continues to be thought of as both psychology dispensed from the media and psychology about the media and its influence. Dr. Phil McGraw (2017), a well-known television personality, is probably the most recent example of the former, and many of the books and articles published at least from the beginning of this 21st century through the present represent a plethora of writings from the latter. Clinical psychologists often define themselves through the therapy they use or the individuals they treat: Cognitive-behavioral therapy, psychodynamic therapy, and family systems therapy are just a few of the more well-known forms. Mental health professionals may even have their titles defined for them; in some states the law influences psychology by dictating which mental health professionals are allowed to call themselves psychologists (e.g., Clinical Psychologists Licensing Act, 2015; Psychology Licensing Law, 2003).

DEFINING FORENSIC PSYCHOLOGY

And that last point brings us to the topic of this book: **forensic psychology**. What's in the name? The simplest definition is probably the least often offered one: Forensic psychology is psychology practiced and/or studied for any legal purpose. It is the study of psychology for, about, and within the law. Media influence seems to have impacted the discipline by narrowing or even misleading general understanding of this field; the psychology part seems to have been omitted. Students and others who are new to the study frequently say they are interested in the "criminal mind," want to become profilers or "expert witnesses," (the criminal mind part), and/or are fascinated with DNA, fingerprinting, and the various other forms of evidence and evidence collection portrayed on television. As a professor and frequent applicant interviewer in a forensic psychology graduate program, I have found that much of my time is spent not only explaining what I do, but also explaining what I (and forensic psychology) do not do.

As for the group that thinks forensic psychology pertains only to the criminal justice system, I try to broaden the understanding of the various other areas of forensic psychology that are so much a part of the field: civil law, family law, and juvenile justice. New students may lack knowledge of the definition of "forensic" and have most likely not yet formulated what it means to be a psychologist. Media, represented most frequently these days by fictional television programming, get the blame for the lack of understanding of the actual roles of DNA, fingerprinting, and other tangible evidence used in law enforcement and the criminal justice system. These laboratory items have nothing to do with the world of psychology—they are evidentiary items produced by the research and investigation of the methods of the physical sciences or what is sometimes referred to as "hard science." Yes, sadly, psychology continues to be referred to as a "soft science" among much of the lay public and certainly among some of those who consider themselves to be "hard" scientists. The more accurate terminology for psychology is "social science," and the fact is that forensic psychology, in particular, is evidence based and rests on a strong scientific foundation (APA, 2011; Psychology, n.d.).

So, for all interested individuals, from the potential students who watch the television shows, to the current undergraduate and graduate students and the general public, this book is written to clarify what forensic psychology is and does. Beginning with the simplest definition for forensic psychology and going on to dissect and explain each of the words that make the specialty unique, the goal is to create a picture of the discipline, whether the reader is already involved in forensic psychology, wants to be involved in some capacity in that world, or is merely interested in understanding it.

Although *Forensic Psychology 101* is not meant to cover the entire subject area with the depth and breadth that this continually growing subject deserves, each of the chapters attempts to explain at least one subtopic that is part of the vast discipline of forensic psychology. As a whole, the book is written first to introduce the discipline to those who have yet to decide on the specifics of a career, being mindful that whatever the label and whatever the age, we are never too old to be introduced to new ideas or to find a new career. This book, then, is offered to help clarify and explain the many roles of a forensic psychologist within the discipline.

BACK TO THE BEGINNING

Because the term "forensic psychology" had to originate somewhere at some time, it seemed appropriate to the title of this chapter to take a historical look back. The *Oxford English Dictionary* (OED; 1989) provides the derivation of "forensic," which can be traced back to 1659. The word is said to have derived from the Latin word for "forum," and was apparently used to describe various types of legal/ courtroom undertakings, such as court pleadings. In giving an example of the word's use as an adjective, the OED disappointingly uses "forensic medicine." However, since multiple searches produced no consensus regarding the first use of the word "psychology," finding a first use of the two words together was obviously not realistic. So, finally giving up on what turned out to be more of a quixotic-like quest than a linguistic one, the search turned to actual application (Cervantes & Grossman, 2003; Simpson, Weiner, & Oxford University Press, 1989).

Psychological Origins

The search for a first application of the term "forensic psychology" finally produced reportable results. As with most psychological inquiries, the results were not linear, but often meandering and even a bit murky. However, although exact dates might be somewhat conflicting, varying from 1893 to 1896, and no doubt he never used the word "forensic," James McKeen Cattell is recognized by most as the first psychologist to combine the law and psychology in his research

7

(i.e., History of Forensic Psychology, 2013; Parrott, 1997). In fact, in 1895, the experimental psychologist Cattell wrote:

> As a last example of the usefulness of measurements of the accuracy of observation and memory I may refer to its application in courts of justice. The probable accuracy of a witness could be measured and his testimony weighed accordingly . . . The testimony could be collected independently, and be given to experts who could affirm for example that the chances are 19 to 1 that the homicide was committed by the defendant . . . (pp. 65–66).

Cattell experimented with the accuracy of the memories of 56 junior psychology students at Columbia University to arrive at this groundbreaking idea. Previously and in contradiction, researchers were of the opinion that "useful applications of the material sciences have no parallel in the case of the mental sciences" (Cattell, 1895, p. 765). Cattell posed a series of both academic and practical questions testing the memories and powers of observation of these 56 students. From their responses, he inferred that individual recollections, when compared and contrasted, were more reliable and valid than were group responses after collaboration. He applied his theory to jury deliberations and concluded that in court, the "independently formed verdict of three jurors if concordant would probably have more validity than the unanimous verdict of 12 jurors in consultation" (Cattell, 1895, p. 76). Unfortunately, his tests were not considered reliable, and James Cattell terminated these experiments (Parrott, 1997).

The fact remains, however, that there does not seem to be an earlier researcher or theorist who addressed the usefulness of psychology, or "mental science" as Cattell called it, in the courtroom. Hugo Munsterberg has been referred to as the "father of forensic psychology" due to the publication of his book, *On the Witness Stand: Essays on Psychology and Crime* (1908), but his work followed Cattell's by at least 12 years (Huss, 2009).

Interestingly, and possibly as the stimulus for further research discussed earlier, both Cattell and Munsterberg studied under Wilhelm Wundt, the "father of experimental psychology," in Leipzig, Germany, before returning to the United States to assume their respective university positions (Boring, 1950). Cattell, born in the United States, left to study under Wundt, who had opened the first psychology laboratory in Leipzig, Germany, sometime between 1875 and 1879 (Boring, 1950; Harper, 1950). Munsterberg, younger than Cattell by 3 years and born in Germany, was also Wundt's student. The students received their doctorates from Wundt 1 year apart, and both returned to the United States to take prestigious positions at major universities. One can only conjecture how Wilhelm Wundt's mentorship influenced his famous students' interest in what we now call forensic psychology.

Legal Origins

Although much more will be said in Chapter 2 about the United States (U.S.) Constitution and the legal system it created, using a case from England as the first case to illustrate this very American discipline might seem odd without a short explanation. Why would a country that fought a war to gain its freedom from a country that was "destructive" of the rights of "Life, Liberty and the pursuit of Happiness," take that country's legal tradition (U.S. Declaration of Independence, 1776, para. 2)? Historically, there are only two major legal traditions: common law and civil law (O'Connor, 2012). England became a common law country in the Middle Ages, while other countries of Europe retained civil law. The main difference between them is that the former bases its legal system on cases and case precedent or judge-made law, while the latter begins with written or codified laws, known as statutes. Presumably, when the first settlers from England came to the American colonies, they brought their familiar legal traditions with them and continued those traditions because they were what they knew (Molina, n.d.). There is no question that the United States remains a common law country, but two and a half centuries later, many state systems are a mixture of common and civil law (Common Law and Civil Law Traditions, n.d.).

In reading through this book, it will become apparent that statutory law often follows judge-made law (common law) in the United States, and just as statutes follow judge-made law, so the law follows psychology. The Amicus Curiae brief filed by the APA in the case of *Hall v. Florida* (2014) in Chapter 4 is an example of the law following psychology.

Tarasoff v. Regents of the University of California (1976) is a precedent-setting example of how case law precedes statutory law in the common law tradition. Briefly, Prosenjit Poddar, a University of California student, sought psychological help from the school's mental health services. During treatment, he told the therapist he was going to kill Tatiana Tarasoff. The therapist told his superiors, who called the police. After investigating, the police released Poddar, but no one told anyone in the Tarasoff family what Poddar had said. Poddar then killed Tatiana Tarasoff, and the Tarsoffs sued the university and all parties involved. The California Supreme Court reversed the lower court's decision to dismiss the case and stated that the therapist owed a duty of reasonable care to protect Tatiana (*Tarasoff v. Regents*, 1976). California and the vast majority of states now have statutes codifying that decision (see e.g., CA Civil Code § 43.92; Reamer, 2016).[2]

So, while Cattell may have been the first to give a specific voice to the potential use of psychology in the courtroom (at least in the United States), in the tradition of the common law, the United States adopted a precedent-setting English case in what was one of the first psychologically based verdicts in a criminal case.

SPOTLIGHT ON CASES

The Queen v. Daniel McNaughton (Bousfield & Merrett, 1843)

The case that best illustrates the beginnings of forensic psychology as we know it, with all its testimony, argument, and verbal analysis, was compiled into a 78-page booklet by a law student and a stenographer who claimed in the Preface that they did so because they knew the case was destined to make new law (Bousfield & Merrett, 1843). All forensic psychology students learn that 52 years before Cattell wrote about the potential use of psychological testimony in the courtroom, Daniel McNaughton decided to kill the Prime Minister of England, Robert Peel. Although he killed Peel's secretary by mistake, McNaughton's defense to the murder charge was that he was being persecuted by the unpopular Prime Minister, could not escape him, and would finally have peace if he killed him (White, 1927). In spite of the fact that McNaughton had traveled from his home in Glasgow, Scotland (where Peel was not), to Peel's home at 10 Downing Street in London (where Peel was) to commit this homicide, the witnesses, the defendant, and the law's application to the facts convinced the jury that McNaughton was insane at the time of the murder and was, therefore, not guilty by reason of insanity.

While the prosecution conceded that the (English) law was such that insanity was an absolute defense to murder, the point was made that several earlier cases, with facts showing odd behavior on the part of the defendants, still resulted in guilty verdicts, and this result should not be different. However, the judge's charge to the jury was very specific in that if all the testimony presented by lay witnesses, the defendant, and many medical experts proved that McNaughton was incapable of "distinguishing between right and wrong," then he was not legally responsible for the death of the victim (Bousfield & Merrett, 1843, p. 74). Interestingly, the judge made very clear to the jury that in his opinion the medical testimony was "on one side and there is no part of it which leaves any doubt in the mind" (Bousfield & Merrett, 1843, p. 74).

Although one might question why this English case became precedent setting for the "not guilty by reason of insanity" plea in the United States, the facts and circumstances of the *Queen v. McNaughton* (1843) provide a near-perfect example from which to begin to understand just how forensic psychology works. In this instance, the construct is insanity—a legal term that requires a legal definition for the courtroom but a scientific explanation, psychological or psychiatric, for its application (Tighe, 2005). The testimony of the medical experts who examined McNaughton provided the application to the individual with their expert knowledge of what James Cattell (1895) called the "mental senses" (p. 765).

The Progeny of McNaughton

Various cases and statutes have been tweaking this definition ever since. While the legal definition of insanity—that is, not knowing the difference between right and wrong—became the **McNaughton Rule**, and is today a recognized plea in the vast majority of American states, there are other definitions utilized in the various states as well (Lilienfeld & Arkowitz, 2011). Interestingly, the American Law Institute added a second prong to the insanity test in 1962 by expanding, in its **Model Penal Code**, the definition of someone who is legally insane (at the time of the commission of the act) to include anyone with a relevant mental defect who could not control his or her behavior; the defect, however, could not be the result of drugs or other substances (Allen, 1962). What is interesting about the date of this amendment is that it was not until that same year that psychologists were even allowed to testify as experts in the courts in the United States (*Jenkins v. United States*, 1962). Prior to the decision in *Jenkins v. United States* (1962), the federal courts had not allowed psychologists to testify as experts because they were not medical doctors. However, in reviewing the lower court's decision not to consider opinion testimony by psychologists regarding the diagnosis of a mental disorder, the court, after going through the rigorous education experienced by doctoral level psychologists stated that "the Ph.D. in Clinical Psychology involves some—and often much—training and experience in the diagnosis and treatment of mental disorders" and concluded that psychologists' testimony could and should be admitted at the discretion of the judge (lines 637 and 638).

So, the roots of forensic psychology are based in the law and psychology. The *McNaughton* court was not playing psychologist when it called the jury's attention to the medical testimony and rendered a judgment of not guilty by reason of insanity. The law could do that because the very definition of the crime required a showing of intent—as was defined by the law. And James McKeen Cattell was not playing at being a lawyer when his experiment convinced him that psychology could be used in the courtroom: Who better to explain how the mind did or did not form the requisite intent?

AND HOW IT GREW: FORENSIC PSYCHOLOGY TODAY

It is the mental health professional, today's forensic psychologist, who provides the testimony that will help the trier of fact, usually the jury, to determine whether a particular individual **is not guilty by reason of insanity**. Despite so much documented interrelated law and psychology history, many writings attribute the origin of the true practice of forensic psychology to a somewhat recent recognition by the APA and its approval of the **Specialty Guidelines for Forensic Psychology**, which were originally adopted in 1991 and frequently revised (APA, 2011). Yet, the over 3,000-member division that has adopted the term and is responsible for the Specialty Guidelines calls itself the **American Psychology-Law Society**, not the Forensic Psychology Division. The much smaller organization (347 members listed) that does bear the specialty's name, the **American Academy of Forensic Psychology** (AAFP), was founded in 1978. The AAFP collaborated with the APA's Division 41 to write and promulgate the original specialty guidelines in 1991 (APA, 2011). In fact, even though law and psychology have been partners who are used to solving problems as partners, it does not appear that there is any real consensus as to when the actual term "forensic psychology" came into general use.

There's little doubt that almost everyone who researches and/ or teaches forensic psychology conceptualizes it somewhat differently. The subtopics and definitions vary and are arranged in multiple permutations depending upon the perspective of the teacher or author. However, the one consistency is the context: Just as the law is studied through the cases that give life to the statutes, forensic psychology is best understood by studying its place in the courts. Since this is true, the question must be asked once again: If we know that "forensic" has to do with the law and/or the courts, and "psychology" has to do with human behavior, does the origin of the term "forensic psychology" and how it is defined really matter (Psychology, n.d.)? The simple answer is yes. The rest of the chapters of this book explain why. For any interested party, the parameters must be defined and understood, and most are not familiar enough with the day-to-day workings of the law and its often inextricable relationship with psychology to fully grasp the methodology, ethics, careers, constructs, and general influence of the specialty and the mental health professionals who work within this specialized discipline—hence, this book.

WHAT TO EXPECT GOING FORWARD

The case of Daniel McNaughton (1843) and the research of James McKeen Cattell (1895) may seem to be unrelated as a practical matter, but together they serve to illustrate a broad foundation and the deep roots of today's practice of forensic psychology. They can also be thought of as the root system from which the remaining eight chapters of this book, possibly to be viewed as the branches, grew (see Figure 1.1). The legal roots are established in Chapter 2 with a description of the relevant parts of the U.S. Constitution. Utilizing the growing tree for the analogy to explain the three branches of government is appropriate—if not very original. The first three articles of the Constitution set the framework for our federal government. With an emphasis on Article III, which establishes the judiciary to interpret the laws, the chapter details the making of federal law. Article I establishes the legislative branch (Congress) which makes the laws, and Article II provides for the executive branch (the President) to enforce the laws. The chapter explains the Tenth Amendment provision that allows for the states to have their own governments, including their own court systems and laws, and how this is all relevant to the practice of forensic psychology.

Forensic psychology can be looked at as applying the relevant psychological constructs to that basic legal understanding, and there are discussion questions and suggestions for further reading to supplement that foundation. Another part of achieving a basic legal understanding is reading and understanding cases. Law students learn how to read and understand cases by "briefing" them, utilizing descriptive captions to find the most important points of a case.

Chapter 3 completes the introductory section of the book, and begins the format that is followed throughout. In addition to giving an overview and explanation of how the chapter topic, behavior and the law, work, at least one relevant and usually United States (U.S.) Supreme Court case that illustrates the constructs in the chapter is presented. In Chapter 3, that is the 2015 case *Elonis v. United States*. Following the case is the first interviewed forensic psychologist, who describes what he does as a county employee. No matter what the topic of a particular chapter, the news always reveals something relevant, and Chapter 3 continues with an "In the News" section that

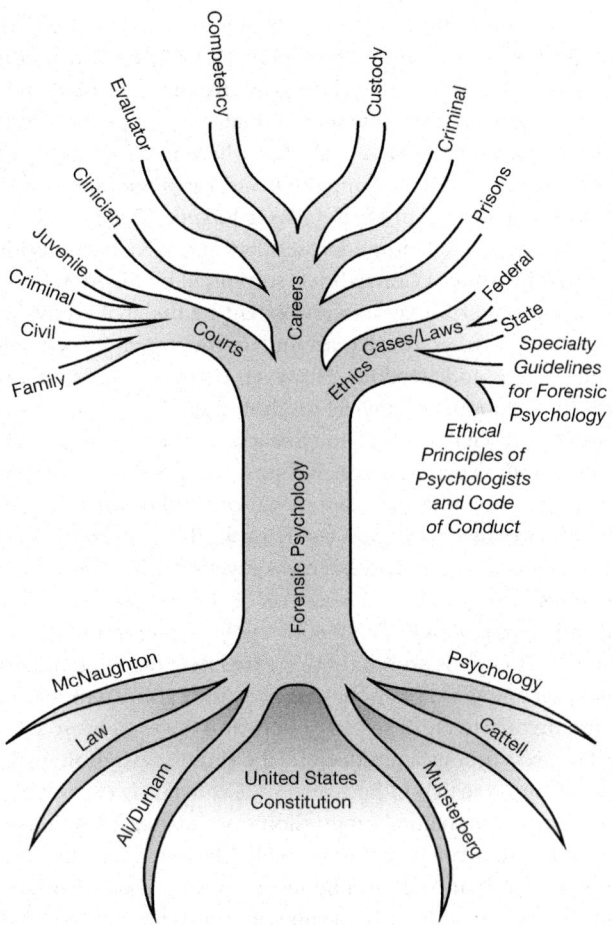

FIGURE 1.1 The growth of forensic psychology.

exemplifies the constructs of context and perception. Again and throughout the remainder of the book, a summary is followed by questions for discussion.

Chapter 4, the first of the four chapters of Part II, begins to explain the specific work of the forensic psychologist in specific legal situations. Chapter 4 takes the reader through a criminal trial, beginning with the crime and investigation, and ending with the sentencing and post-trial motions and appeals. Along the route of the trial, the various junctures that require the expertise of a forensic psychologist are explored. Two forensic psychologists give their personal and professional insights as a sex offender evaluator and a prison psychologist. Because criminal law is that area where freedom and life can often be at issue, two U.S. Supreme Court cases relevant to forensic psychology practice are briefed. *Atkins v. Virginia* (2002) and *Roper v. Simmons* (2005) were landmark cases that may have been decided at least in part by Amicus Curiae briefs submitted by the APA.

While Chapter 5 may to some extent be the civil equivalent of Chapter 4, the issues revolve around money and property rather than life, death, and freedom. However, there are no fewer opportunities for the input of forensic psychologists. Civil matters include torts which are civil wrongs and breach of contract suits. Witness testimony, both expert and eye, and jury selection can be important factors in the outcome of a case. A nationally known forensic psychologist shares his experiences testifying for the defense and plaintiff in employment cases, and several cases covering rules of admissibility of expert testimony and various aspects of civil matters are presented.

Family court matters are the subject of Chapter 6, and the changing family structure is seen to have created new fields of practice for forensic psychologists. From the case presented about a modern marriage and divorce to child custody issues and the even more sobering subject of "psychological autopsies," the forensic psychologist's role in practice and research in family court is constantly expanding.

As a somewhat natural progression from matters of child custody and teen suicide, Part II concludes with Chapter 7 and the forensic psychologist's role in the juvenile justice system. Two main areas of juvenile justice are addressed. Keeping in mind that the "best interest of the child" is the overarching policy of the courts, the areas are easily divided into that which happens to the child and that which the child makes happen. In the first category are education and care (see, for example, CA Welfare & Institutions Code § 300, 1937; *Larry P. v. Riles,* 1979). All children are entitled to a free and public education and to care and protection by their parents (or the state if necessary; Education for All Handicapped Children Act, 1975). Then there are the children who are categorized as delinquent, those children whose acts are status infractions such as breaking curfew or truancy and those children whose acts would be crimes if they were adults (see, for example, CA Welfare & Institutions Code §§ 601 & 602, 1937). A forensic psychologist who specializes in the legal problems of at-risk children shares his experience in evaluating and treating these children.

The last two chapters make up Part III, Reconciling the Disciplines. The disciplines referred to are those of the forensic psychologist and the attorney. They must work closely together, but there can be conflict regarding the specific roles of each during the course of a case. Although Chapter 8 follows a similar format as the previous chapters, it deviates in that two attorneys share their experiences in working with forensic psychologists. These attorneys were chosen for their specialties; one is a criminal defense attorney, and the other is a family law certified specialist. As will be seen, these are the two legal areas that employ forensic psychologists on the most regular bases.

All chapters lead to Chapter 9. The growth of forensic psychology is explored in a very recent case regarding the influence of the APA. It also illustrates how the U.S. Supreme Court depends and expands upon precedent. Relevant newspaper articles are so frequent that supplements could continually be added. While Chapter 9 is the final chapter of *Forensic Psychology 101*, the goal is that it will serve as the first chapter in a very rewarding career.

SUMMARY

This first introductory chapter began with an overview of the various types of psychology and psychology practice. With that background, the focus was narrowed to forensic psychology, including its origins and application. The origin of the science was traced to legal and psychological roots that began not only separately but in two (maybe three) different countries, then came together somehow to form one inextricable discipline, and branched out to encompass almost all, if not all, aspects of the two disciplines at its foundation: psychology and the law. In describing the origins and the evolution of forensic psychology, the work of James Cattell, who was among the first to experiment with the use of psychology in the courtroom, and the case that gave us the McNaughton Rule were described. To explain why the *Queen v. McNaughton* (1843) case has such historic relevance, some background regarding the United States' use of the common law tradition from England was presented. An overview of the topics and format found in the remainder of the book was also provided.

DISCUSSION QUESTIONS

1. Although *Tarasoff v. Regents of the University of California* (1976) was a California case and did not have to be followed in other states, most states did enact some form of a *Tarasoff* law. Discuss why this case might have had such a far-reaching effect. You can find the case by using Google or another search engine: *Tarasoff v. Regents of University of California* 17 Cal.3d 425 (1976).
2. It is important to understand that the word "forensic" is merely a descriptor. Why do you think this is so?
3. There are many constructs that lend themselves to both psychological and legal research or even psycholegal research. Privacy is one of those constructs (as you will see in Chapter 2). Can you think of two or three others?
4. From this brief background provided in the chapter, what do you think would be the most interesting area of forensic psychology to work in?

NOTES

1. Some states restrict the title of psychologist to licensed individuals. Although forensic psychologists (people who have a background and/ or degree in forensic psychology) may devote their professional time to academia and/or research, they cannot ethically call themselves psychologists according to the California, Illinois, and some other Boards of Psychology. In the interest of full disclosure, then, even though I am a licensed attorney and have a doctorate in psychology, because I am not licensed to practice psychology, I am an attorney and media psychologist.
2. In 2013, California amended its *Tarasoff* statute to eliminate the duty to warn. Some state statutes have both duties, some have one or the other, and some do not make the duty mandatory (See CA Civil Code §43.92).

REFERENCES

Allen, F. A. (1962). Article 3: The rule of the American Law Institute's Model Penal Code. *Marquette Law Review*, *45*(4), 494–505.

American Psychological Association (APA). (n.d.). Society for media psychology and technology. Retrieved from http://www.apa.org/about/division/div46.aspx

American Psychological Association (APA). (2011). *Specialty guidelines for forensic psychology*. Washington, DC: Author (*American Psychologist*, 2013, 68(1), 7–19. doi:10.1037/a0029889).

Boring, E. G. (1950). *A history of experimental psychology* (2nd ed.). Englewood Cliffs, NJ: Prentice-Hall.

Bousfield, R. M., & Merrett, R. (1843). *Report of the trial of Daniel M'Naughton at the Central Criminal court*. London, UK: Henry Renshaw.

CA Welfare & Institutions Code §§ 300, 601, 602 (1937).

Cattell, J. M. (1895). Measurements of the accuracy of recollection. *Science*, *2*(49), 761–766. Retrieved from https://www.jstor.org/stable/1623733?seq=1#page_scan_tab_contents

Cervantes, S. M., & Grossman, E. (2003). *Don Quixote*. New York, NY: Ecco. Retrieved from https://www.amazon.com/Don-Quixote-Miguel-Cervantes-ebook/dp/B001R1LCKS

Clinical Psychologists Licensing Act, IL 225ILCS § 3 (2015).

Common law and civil law traditions. (n.d.). Robbins Collection, School of Law, Boalt Hall. Retrieved from https://www.law.berkeley.edu/library/robbins/CommonLawCivilLawTraditions.html

Education for All Handicapped Children Act, PL 94–142 (1975).

Ferguson, C. J. (2016). *Media psychology 101*. New York, NY: Springer.

Harper, R. S. (1950). The first psychological laboratory. *Isis*, *41*(2), 158–161. Retrieved from http://www.journals.uchicago.edu/doi/citedby/10.1086/349141

History of Forensic Psychology. (2013). Psychology educator. Retrieved from https://psychologyeducator.wordpress.com/2013/09/04/the-history-of-forensic-psychology/

Huss, M. T. (2009). *Forensic psychology: Research, clinical practice, and applications*. West Sussex, UK: Wiley-Blackwell.

Larry P. v. Riles 495 F. Supp. 926 (ND Cal. 1979).

Lilienfeld, S. O., & Arkowitz, H. (2011, January). The insanity verdict on trial. *Scientific American*. Retrieved from https://www.scientificamerican.com/article/the-insanity-verdict-on-trial

Molina, S. E. (n.d.). Roots of our legal system: The foundation for growth. American Bar Association. Retrieved from https://www.americanbar

.org/publications/tyl/topics/legal-history/roots-our-legal-system-foundation-growth.html

O'Connor, V. (2012). *Common law and civil law traditions.* INPROL—International Network to Promote the Rule of Law. Retrieved from https://www.fjc.gov/sites/default/files/2015/Common%20and%20Civil%20Law%20Traditions.pdf

Parrott, B. (1997). *James McKeen Cattell.* Retrieved from http://www.muskingum.edu/~psych/psycweb/history/cattell.htm

Phil, M. (2017). *About Dr. Phil.* Retrieved from https://www.drphil.com/about-dr-phil/

Popper, K. (2002). *The logic of scientific discovery.* New York, NY: Routledge Classics.

Psychology. (n.d.). *Oxford Dicionaries.com.* Retrieved from https://en.oxforddictionaries.com/definition/psychology

Psychology Licensing Law, CA Business & Professions Code § 2903 (2003).

Reamer, F. G. (2016, May). The duty and privilege to warn and protect. *Social Work Today.* Retrieved from http://www.socialworktoday.com/news/eoe_0516.shtml

Simpson, J. A., Weiner, E. S. C., & Oxford University Press. (1989). *Oxford English dictionary.* Oxford, UK: Clarendon Press.

Tarasoff v. Regents of the University of California, 131 Cal. Rptr. 14 (Cal. 1976).

Tighe, J. A. (2005). What's in a name? *Journal of the American Academy of Psychiatry and the Law, 33*(2), 252–258.

U.S. Declaration of Independence, para. 2 (1776).

White, A. M. (1927). Legal insanity in criminal cases past, present and future. *Journal of Criminal Law and Criminology, 18*(2), 165–174. Retrieved from http://scholarlycommons.law.northwestern.edu/cgi/viewcontent.cgi?article=2053&context=jclc

Constitutional Law and What Forensic Psychologists Need to Know

OVERVIEW

This chapter was originally titled Law School 101. The title seemed fitting in that trying to understand the roots of forensic psychology without understanding the roots of our legal system would most likely result in not understanding forensic psychology and its application. However, because the goal is actually to understand and be able to apply the law in the context of psychology, getting directly to the source is much more efficient. Another problem with that title arises from experience. Rarely, if at all, throughout my own experience as a law student, as a law school professor at several institutions, and in talking to alumni from a large number of law schools throughout the country have I heard fond reminiscing about the law school experience. While, as is seen later in this chapter, the most common law school teaching method is quite effective, the students who received it do not generally miss their law school days. Chapter titles and education of future attorneys aside, however, in 1989, Michael Hoeflich, in attempting to explain why legal education needed to be expanded beyond law schools, wrote:

> We must teach everyone, whatever their field of study, about basic constitutional law and regulation, for only then can they fully and knowingly participate in our constitutional government structures. . . . It needs to be taught to undergraduates, to high school students, to elementary school students. And it needs to be taught to all of them, from sixth graders to law students . . . as a complex part of human social organization with a history and a broad social and cultural purpose. (pp. 796–797)

Unfortunately, although a laudable goal, this type of education does not yet seem to universally exist. From my experience and that of others who have taught them, even first-year law students have had very little exposure to the **United States (U.S.) Constitution**; almost none have previously read it in its entirety, and many express surprise at its brevity when they do. Recently, the successful presidential candidate from a major political party was accused by a naturalized citizen of not having read the Constitution; to the best of my recollection the accusation was never rebutted, and within the first 100 days of his inauguration, at least one of his **executive orders** underwent and lost a **constitutional challenge** (Jarrett, 2017). Further, although it is said the power to make an executive order is derived from the Constitution, the Constitution does not expressly state the president has such executive power (see Article II, § 2; Chu & Garvey, 2014). As seen later in this chapter, as well as throughout any constitutional discussion, much of the intent of the Founding Fathers is subject to modern interpretation. The document that provides the foundation for this country's entire legal system, not to mention the governmental structure, and many social constructs, is composed of a short Preamble, seven articles, and 27 amendments—yet it is a rare individual who reads the Constitution without the impetus of an assignment.

SOME RELEVANT CONSTITUTIONAL CONTENT

An understanding of the contents of at least the first three of those articles and a few of the amendments is imperative for an appreciation of how the law works, which in turn is critical for those who would be working with, for, and in legal environments. For example, law students learn during their first year of study that invasion of privacy is a tort, or civil wrong, for which there is a legal remedy if all elements of the tort are proved to be present. They learn this initially from a United States (U.S.) Supreme Court case that in 1965 proclaimed that the **U.S. Constitution's Bill of Rights** (first 10 Amendments), although never mentioning the word, guarantees individual privacy through "penumbras," or emanations from those rights that actually are specified (*Griswold v. Connecticut*). While this might be a first exposure to constitutional interpretation, to understand how the Supreme Court arrived at that conclusion without explicit language, the education must start at the beginning. In fact, an understanding of how the case arrived at the U.S. Supreme Court initially is the true beginning.

Article I of the U.S. Constitution provides for a **legislative branch** consisting of two houses, the **Senate** and the **House of Representatives**, that together are called Congress and have the power and duty to enact all federal **statutory** laws.[1] With two senators from each of 50 states, and representatives based on population, Congress consists of 100 senators and 435 representatives, for a total of 535 members.[2]

The congressionally enacted laws are presumed to be constitutional unless challenged in court and proven not to be so. **Article II** creates an **executive branch** of government, a **President**, and a **Vice President** with broadly stated duties and obligations that are primarily meant to enforce the laws enacted by Congress. Aside from being the **commander-in-chief of the Armed Forces**, the President appoints a **Cabinet**, the agencies created under the various

Cabinet departments, and other advisors as part of his or her White House staff (U.S. Const., art. II § 2).[3] It is from the second section of this article that the President's executive privilege power is said to have originated (Chu & Garvey, 2014; Newland, 2015). **Article III** establishes a judicial branch of government, the branch that interprets the laws enacted by Congress and enforced by the President. As has already been seen and is repeated throughout, the judiciary takes its power of interpretation very seriously, and it is from this power that we get our other type of law: the **common law**, or more literally **case law** or **judge-made law**. The very first sentence of Article III states that the "judicial Power of the United States, shall be vested on one supreme Court, and in such inferior Courts as the Congress may from time to time ordain and establish" (U.S. Const., § 1, 1789).

The Federal Judiciary

To establish those federal courts (and implement the U.S. Supreme Court), Congress needed to enact one of our first federal statutes, commonly referred to as the **Judiciary Act of 1789**. This was the same year the U.S. Constitution was ratified by the 13 new states, and 2 years before the states ratified what we know as the Bill of Rights.[4] The "inferior" federal courts Congress established with that legislation began with the federal district courts (§ 3)—that is, the trial courts that hear both civil and criminal matters that either arise out of federal laws, the U.S. Constitution, or parties from different states (28 U.S.C. §§ 1331 & 1332; Gomberg, circa 1990). Today, there are **94 judicial districts** in the United States, including the District of Columbia, Puerto Rico, the Virgin Islands, Guam, and the Northern Mariana Islands, with at least one district in each of the 50 states. The next level of judicial review established by the Judiciary Act is the **Circuit Courts of Appeal** (§ 4); the 94 districts are reduced to13 circuits, 12 regional courts, and one court with federal jurisdiction. This last court also hears appeals from federal administrative agencies.

The highest court, of course, is the U.S. Supreme Court, which has quite limited **jurisdiction** (power) and, for a variety of reasons, hears far fewer cases than the other courts (C-SPAN, 2009; Gomberg, circa 1990). When interviewed for C-SPAN's Supreme Court Project in 2009, Associate Justice Stephen Breyer told the interviewer that of approximately 80,000 potential cases, the Supreme Court receives

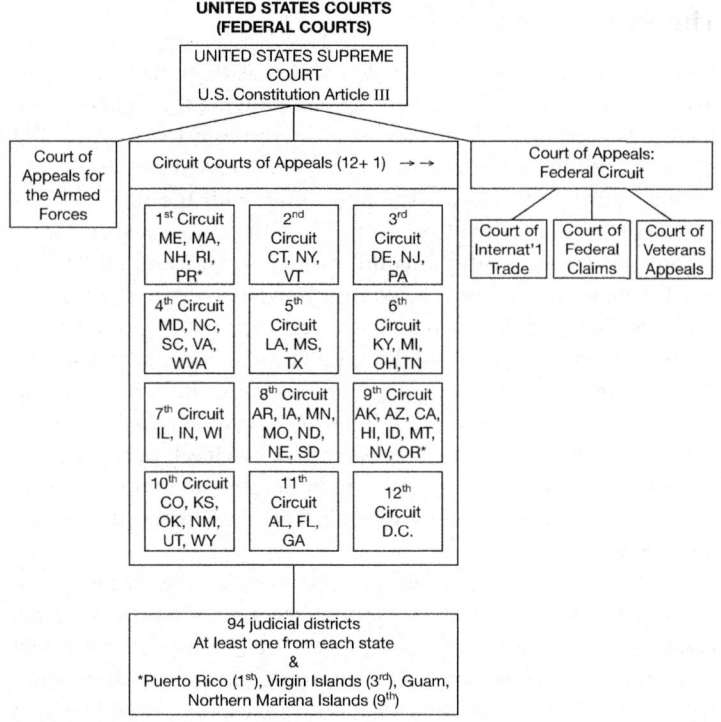

**UNITED STATES COURTS
(FEDERAL COURTS)**

UNITED STATES SUPREME
COURT
U.S. Constitution Article III

Court of
Appeals for
the Armed
Forces

Circuit Courts of Appeals (12+ 1) → →

Court of Appeals:
Federal Circuit

1st Circuit ME, MA, NH, RI, PR*	2nd Circuit CT, NY, VT	3rd Circuit DE, NJ, PA
4th Circuit MD, NC, SC, VA, WVA	5th Circuit LA, MS, TX	6th Circuit KY, MI, OH,TN
7th Circuit IL, IN, WI	8th Circuit AR, IA, MN, MO, ND, NE, SD	9th Circuit AK, AZ, CA, HI, ID, MT, NV, OR*
10th Circuit CO, KS, OK, NM, UT, WY	11th Circuit AL, FL, GA	12th Circuit D.C.

Court of
Internat'l
Trade

Court of
Federal
Claims

Court of
Veterans
Appeals

94 judicial districts
At least one from each state
&
*Puerto Rico (1st), Virgin Islands (3rd), Guam,
Northern Mariana Islands (9th)

FIGURE 2.1 U.S. courts (federal courts).

about 8,000 requests each session and actually hears about 80 to 100 of those (see Figure 2.1).

The various trial courts and circuit courts of appeal from which most of the cases come are located within the districts and circuits they represent, which means they often sit next to or even within the same complex as do state courts, which operate under entirely separate systems. The physical location of the court is called the **venue**, and is where the case is actually heard; venue is based on the convenience of the parties. This is separate from the jurisdiction, which is the court's power to render a valid decision. It should also be noted that these federal courts, under certain circumstances, might base their substantive decisions on the laws of the states in which they sit (see e.g., *Erie Railroad Co. v. Tompkins*, 1938; Federal Rules of Civil Procedure, 2016).

to have a long history and much dedicated research in both fields (Gomberg, 2012). Using the privacy construct as it was discussed in the case of *Griswold v. Connecticut* (1965) might help illustrate the workings of both a state system and the federal system, as well as how the dually researched construct presented psychological issues with which the Court grappled. By way of introduction, some specific and general information regarding that case in particular and a method for reading cases that is beneficial for forensic psychology students follows.

First, a simplified version of the judicial history of that landmark U.S. Supreme Court case involves almost every court level: Griswold, an executive with Planned Parenthood, was arrested and convicted in the Connecticut state trial court under an 1879 Connecticut state law that prohibited advising married (or not) couples about contraception. She appealed the conviction to the Appellate Division of the Circuit Court (of Connecticut), lost that appeal, and appealed again to the highest court in the state, the Supreme Court of Errors, where she again lost. The basis of her appeals was that the state law under which she was convicted violated the **Due Process Clause of the Fourteenth Amendment** of the U.S. Constitution. Although more will be said about the substantive issues of the case later (as well as the Due Process Clause), what is important here is that because this case challenged a state law's constitutionality and had exhausted the state court's jurisdiction, the U.S. Supreme Court could hear it and make a final decision on the constitutionality of the state law (C-SPAN, 2009; *Griswold v. Connecticut*, 1965).

More generally, because understanding cases is an integral part of the work of a forensic psychologist, learning to read them for a particular purpose in the same way law students do is both efficient and effective. Law students generally learn the law through the case-book method first developed for Harvard law students by the then dean of the law school, Christopher Columbus Langdell, during the 1870s (Garvin, 2003). Law students read mostly landmark cases or at least cases that are included in their assigned reading to make a particular legal point. They "brief" the cases with the purpose of finding the relevant components so as to understand the significance of the case. This is not as easy as it sounds, as not all judges (or their clerks) write either clearly or succinctly, and the task of the law student is to wade through the verbiage and find, among other things, the facts the court needed to make a decision, what law/rule was at issue, and how that rule was applied to the issue raised by the facts of the particular case and used to render a judgment, often in the form of a new or modified rule (Delaney, 2011). **Student briefs**, which are basically focused summaries, are different from **attorney briefs** that present a case to the courts. The latter are formal documents that are written within the rules of a particular court's requirements, advocating a position on a particular topic for the court's consideration.

Reading a Case

Cases are read for a purpose. Attorneys become quite skilled at perusing cases to find the important points relevant to their needs. Law students learn by reading and discussing how laws were applied to facts and debated until a jury or judge reached a conclusion. Almost all the cases that are read for briefing are from at least an appeals level. Because of that, the facts are usually not in dispute; the ultimate facts have been determined in the lower court. On appeal, the question is the application of those facts to a law or about the law itself.

The Parties

At the outset, understanding who's suing whom for what can be a bit complicated but does make the reading easier. The aggrieved party is the **plaintiff** in civil cases and the **prosecution** in criminal matters. Usually that is the first name seen in a suit at the trial or first level of litigation. Although almost always a person or persons in a civil matter, the plaintiff might also be the name of a company, agency, or government entity. In criminal matters, this is not the case. Crimes are acts against society, so the society that has been harmed has representatives who prosecute the case as the plaintiff. This can be a city, county, state, the United States, or any legally sanctioned government office, depending upon which law is determined to have been broken. Whether the case is civil or criminal, the individual or entity being sued is the **defendant**.

There are, however, cases in which there is no aggrieved party, merely individuals who need or want to go to court to ask for the court's opinion or decision about a matter. Nobody feels harmed or aggrieved, and there may not even be another party involved. When that person or entity comes into the court, he or she is a **petitioner**. If there is another party, the reference is to a **respondent**. However, just to make matters a little murkier and more complicated, these terms also refer to parties coming before the U.S. Supreme Court for a decision. No matter who was the aggrieved party in the lower court, the party asking the Supreme Court for its decision is the petitioner—whether it is a civil or criminal matter. And just to complete the possibility of party identifiers, when either party is unhappy with the decision of a trial court in civil matters or the defendant loses in a criminal matter, those people can appeal the lower court decision if they can find a legal reason to do so. In such a case, the unhappy party is called the **appellant**, and the lower court winner is the **appellee**.

The Place(s)

So, when reading a case, the names of individuals versus individuals will usually signify civil matters; when "the State," "the People," or "the United States" is a named party, the case is usually criminal. When there are no truly legally aggrieved parties, there might be only a single name referred to as "In re" or the "Matter of . . . ." Finally, dates and places are important in case law. Therefore, being able to understand the case citation matters. Although in this age we are able to find almost any sort of information within seconds on an electronic device, cases are and have been recorded in books. Every case that has been reported will have a citation that contains the name of the case, where it can be found (the particular volumes and the page number), and in what year it was decided.

Taking that explanation into consideration, what follows is what could have been a very brief student brief presented here to make several points about the law and to illustrate the explanations provided previously. The headings are those commonly used by law students when reporting a case for discussion.

SPOTLIGHT ON CASES

Griswold v. Connecticut, 381 U.S. 479 (1965)

The title and citation provide a lot of information: This 1965 decision, which was written by one but represents the opinion of a majority of U.S. Supreme Court justices, can be found in the official U.S. Supreme Court reports (U.S.) in volume 381, beginning on page 479.

Parties and History: Appellants/petitioners (losers in the lower court): Estelle Griswold (Executive Director) and Dr. C. Lee Buxton (physician/Medical Director) as employees of Planned Parenthood League of Connecticut were arrested and convicted under a Connecticut statute criminalizing the dissemination of birth control. This case was *Connecticut v. Griswold* (1964) (*Griswold v. Connecticut*, 1965). They appealed through the state courts and are appealing the conviction to the U.S. Supreme Court, claiming that the Connecticut law is unconstitutional. Appellee/respondent: The State of Connecticut.

Facts: The appellant/petitioners provided birth control devices and advice to married couples in the course of their professional dealings with those couples through Planned Parenthood. The statutes provide that persons who do so are as guilty as those who utilize the birth control, and they were fined $100 each.

Issue: The issue presents a Constitutional argument: Do the statutes banning the use of contraception and the assistance with or dissemination of contraception violate the Due Process Clause of the Fourteenth Amendment, which prohibits states from enacting laws that do not give citizens the rights of legal due process granted by the U.S. Constitution? Simply stated:

Is the Connecticut statute constitutional? More specifically, does a law that intrudes into the bedroom of a married couple and their doctor–patient relationship (traditionally private) violate the Due Process Clause of the Fourteenth Amendment?

Holding: The Connecticut law, "in forbidding the use of contraceptives rather than regulating their manufacture or sale, seeks to achieve its goals by means having a maximum destructive impact upon" a relationship lying within the "zone of privacy, created by several fundamental constitutional guarantees" (*Griswold v. Connecticut*,

Majority Opinion, para. 15). The statutes are overbroad, invade the privacy of marriage, and, therefore, violate several amendments as well as the Fourteenth Amendment, which prevents states from enacting laws that do not allow for due process and equal protection.

Judgment: Reversed for appellant/petitioners.

(Note that while seven justices voted for reversal, three of those did not join in the majority opinion. They **concurred** with the result, but did not agree with the reasoning. Two justices **dissented**. stating that while they did not like the law, it was not unconstitutional.)

Now for the points to be made from this one case: At issue in *Griswold v. Connecticut* (1965) was a statute, a legislatively enacted law. All states have legislatures that enact the laws of those states, while federal laws or statutes are products of Congress. The power to enact these laws comes from the federal and the state constitutions. The second point is that this and all cases illustrate another kind of law that is steeped in the tradition of the English legal system from which it came and upon which U.S. law is based. The common law is the case law that arises from decisions of the judiciary. Traditionally, common law is based on precedent, the cases that came before, wherein the facts, rules, and/or issues may either have an impact on the present case or distinguish the earlier case from the present case. In *Griswold v. Connecticut* (1965), dozens of cases were cited that created precedent for the decision reached in that case. In turn, *Griswold* established the precedent that a law that invaded the privacy of marriage would be considered unconstitutional. Of course, the case arising from a new set of facts on which that new law would be tested would have to show that such a law did invade that marital privacy.

The case of *Griswold v. Connecticut* (1965) represents the zeitgeist of the State of Connecticut and much of the United States through the middle of the 20th century (Revisiting a landmark, 2015). Connecticut was a Catholic state, and the women's movement was in full gear (Walsh, 2010). The legalization of birth control by the U.S. Supreme Court was said to have a major psychological effect on women with regard to their decision-making power and to have impacted our society in general by legally recognizing the individual's right to a "zone of privacy" that had been propounded not only by the law but also by psychologists in other contexts (Fact Sheet, 2000; Confidentiality . . . , 2002).

The ruling in *Griswold v. Connecticut* gave rise to societal changes and became the impetus (amid the development of sophisticated electronic communications) for a plethora of statutory privacy laws (Cline, 2016). Although the psychology of privacy had been recognized as early as 1950 by Maslow, it took the law and the "penumbras" of the Bill of Rights more than a decade to catch up.

UNDERSTANDING THE SYSTEM

Finally, for the sake of completion and clarity of this very short "course," one final distinction needs to be made. Aside from being divided into constitutional, statutory, and common law; federal as well as state laws; and varying levels of courts, as was mentioned earlier and in Chapter 1, our legal system is further divided into civil and criminal law as well as family, probate, and juvenile justice law. Civil laws and lawsuits encompass wrongs against private individuals and entities, be it their persons or property. When those private individuals or entities feel they have been legally injured, they become plaintiffs in lawsuits, and the people they feel have injured them are the defendants. Although there are other types of civil lawsuits (i.e., breach of contract), those types of wrongs are called torts, and they come in three main varieties: intentional torts, negligence, and torts of strict liability.

Civil Courts

Civil wrongs are further divided into torts against the person and torts against property. For example, assault, battery, and false imprisonment are three intentional torts, each having its own distinct elements. The intentional element exists because the perpetrator meant to touch, scare, or restrain the victim depending on the tort being claimed. Negligence is best exemplified by the common professional malpractice or even product liability cases. The perpetrator did not mean to harm the plaintiff, but by breaching a duty of due care and causing damage that was or should have been foreseeable from the act, the defendant can be shown to be the cause of the plaintiff's injuries. Strict liability torts exist as what is sometimes referred to as a "legal fiction." Somebody was hurt; someone else must have been responsible, so that someone else is held liable.

In torts, **the burden of proof** is on the plaintiff to show that the defendant is liable by a "preponderance of the evidence," which is usually described as the majority or most of the evidence. The complaining or injured party, the plaintiff, is compensated by monetary or in-kind damages when he or she proves the case. Sometimes, the defendant, the perpetrator, is merely made to stop doing the damage if the circumstances warrant such a decision. As will be explained in Chapter 3, in civil cases, all interpretations are viewed through the perceptions of the plaintiff.

Criminal Courts

Criminal laws and lawsuits arise from wrongs against society. Even though in most cases, the crime is actually perpetrated against an individual by an individual, the state prosecutes that defendant through its representative, a district or state attorney. Crimes harm all society. The state is the prosecutor, and the accused is the defendant. The punishment can be a fine, jail, prison, probation, a combination depending upon the severity of the crime, or even death. Crimes are further divided into misdemeanors and felonies, with felonies being the more severe and most often punishable with prison terms. To convict a criminal defendant, the prosecutor has the burden of proving the defendant is **"guilty beyond a reasonable doubt."**

All criminal cases are interpreted through the **intent of the defendant**; the **mens rea** or guilty mind is what is at issue, along with the **actus reus**, the act that constitutes the crime. Again, the burden cannot be specifically defined, but it can be looked at through the defense attorney's argument and interpreted in the best light for the defendant. It is the role of the defense attorney to put that reasonable doubt into the minds of the jurors, to suggest that it is reasonable to believe from the evidence that the defendant was not the perpetrator, and did not have or could not form the requisite intent (see Chapter 8).

Equity Courts

Then there are **family, probate,** and **juvenile justice matters**. These three areas are usually considered equitable, requiring equitable decisions rather than strictly legal decisions. Juries are not empaneled for cases in equity, and the decisions are made by a judge. By way of explanation, one example of an equitable family law proceeding would be child custody matters. The law says custody is to be granted "in the best interest of the child" (CA Family Code § 3011, 1993), and guidelines are provided; however, the decision-making responsibility rests with the judge after all the information and evidence is evaluated (see Chapters 6 and 8). Probate matters are similar. They may take the form of distribution of estates, conservatorships, and guardianships, to name just a few matters that probate judges hear. Juvenile justice is a hybrid in that it is neither civil nor criminal, and it is probably the system that is most fluid in a majority of states. In all three of these types of proceedings, the judge "balances the equities" when making a decision.

Family law, probate, and juvenile justice, each of which deserves scrutiny on its own and has its own chapter later in this book, are all governed by individual state law. However, as will be seen, the states cannot be in conflict with the federal law, and sometimes the federal law will change because of the changes among the states. Further, because of the fluidity and subject matter of these areas, forensic psychology almost defines itself when understanding exactly how these types of legal proceedings work.

IN THE NEWS

On April 10, 2017, Neil M. Gorsuch was sworn in as the 113th justice to serve on the U.S. Supreme Court (Davis, 2017). While not specifically relevant to the work of a forensic psychologist, the event is most relevant to any discussion about the Court, particularly when the case under discussion is one in which the majority found such a construct as "privacy," though never specifically mentioned, "emanating" from the rights granted in the first 10 Amendments to the Constitution. Justice

Gorsuch is an "originalist," or strict constructionist (Chemerinsky, 2017). Supreme Court justices are supposedly apolitical, but the reality is that they are nominated by the President and confirmed by the Senate, two branches of our government that are overtly political (U.S. Constitution, Article III, 1789). What the label means is that Justice Gorsuch, as did Justice Antonin Scalia before him, will most likely not engage in finding potential subtleties or possible hidden meanings in the words of the Founding Fathers. He will be a justice who will make his decisions based on what lawyers call the "four corners" of the Constitution. He most likely will not, as do some of his colleagues, go to great lengths to theorize what the Founding Fathers meant; he will not, it is believed, engage in a lot of interpretation (Chemerinsky, 2017).

SUMMARY

In continuing with the themes of Part I, this chapter explained the basic constitutional and legal concepts with which forensic psychologists need to become familiar. Just as lawyers need to have an understanding of the derivation of the law and the powers granted by the U.S. Constitution, so do the members of other professions that work within the courts. Whether the matters are criminal or civil, family or juvenile, forensic psychology can be defined as work in, of, and for the courts (Bartol & Bartol, 2015).

Griswold v. Connecticut (1965) was briefed and explained for several reasons. Aside from the rich judicial history the case revealed, the subject matter was privacy, a crossover construct from psychology and the law that seven members of the Supreme Court found to be implicit within the first 10 Amendments, the Bill of Rights, of the U.S. Constitution. This case also illustrates how a case can move through the state to the federal systems and eventually get to the U.S. Supreme Court. Finally, the case was used to explain the process of case briefing, which will be seen throughout these chapters. Even more relevant for a case that as of this writing is 52 years old, is to look at the most recent (2017) appointee on the Court, and with an understanding of the way in which the U.S. Supreme Court does its work, to follow his opinions as his years of service pass.

DISCUSSION QUESTIONS AND FURTHER READING

1. To get the full impact of the U.S. Constitution, read it in its entirety at https://constitutioncenter.org/media/files/constitution.pdf and think about the following:
   - **Article IV** contains the Full Faith and Credit clause. What does that mean?
   - **Article V** describes the method for amending the Constitution. For decades, both before and after the Civil Rights Act of 1964, the women's movement made strong efforts to pass a Women's Rights Amendment. Why do you think those efforts failed?
   - **Article VI** is titled Debts, Supremacy, Oaths. It states that no government employee will be subjected to a religious test. Many of our presidents have invoked "God" while taking the oath of office. Can you find a reference to God anywhere in the Constitution?
   - Are you surprised by any of the provisions of the Constitution? Do you find it difficult to understand?

2. *Griswold v. Connecticut* (1965) was one of the first cases addressing privacy among consenting adults that the U.S. Supreme Court decided. It was followed by *Eisenstadt v. Baird* (1972), *Bowers v. Hardwick* (1986), and *Lawrence v. Texas* (2003). These cases and/or their briefs or summaries are easily found on the Internet. Discuss the main points of the cases and how the law of privacy evolved behind what we know to be the psychology of privacy. Why do you think it took the Supreme Court 17 years to reverse itself from *Bowers* to *Lawrence*?

NOTES

1. Article I specifies that each state will elect two senators. The number of representatives depends on the state's population.
2. Although the U.S. territories do not have senators, each has one delegate elected to the House of Representatives, as does the District of Columbia (Washington, D.C.) (see Figure 2.1).

3. As of 2017, there were 15 Cabinet departments. The U.S. Vice President is also a member of the Cabinet.
4. Only nine of the new states were required to agree for the new Constitution to be ratified.
5. States have small claims courts where the parties usually represent themselves for civil matters involving small amounts of money, traffic courts for contested traffic infractions, and so on.

REFERENCES

28 U.S.C. §§ 1331, 1332 (1940).

Bartol, C. R., & Bartol, A. M. (2015). *Introduction to forensic psychology: Research and application* (4th ed.). Thousand Oaks, CA: Sage.

California Family Code. (1993). § 3011. Retrieved from https://leginfo.legislature.ca.gov/faces/codes_displaySection.xhtml?sectionNum=3011.&lawCode=FAM

Chemerinsky, E. (2017, February 1). Scalia, the sequel. *The American Prospect.* Retrieved from http://prospect.org/authors/erwin-chemerinsky

Chu, V. S. & Garvey, T. (2014). *Executive orders: Issuance, modification, and revocation.* Congressional Research Service 7-5700. Retrieved from https://fas.org/sgp/crs/misc/RS20846.pdf

Cline, A. (2016). Supreme Court decisions on privacy: *Griswold v. Connecticut. ThoughtCo.* Retrieved from https://www.thoughtco.com/decisions-on-privacy-griswold-v-connecticut-4070860

Confidentiality in the treatment of adolescents. (2002, March). *Monitor on Psychology, 33*(3). Retrieved from http://www.apa.org/education/ce/ethicsrounds400.pdf

C-SPAN (Producer). (2009, June 17). *The Supreme Court project interview with Justice Stephen Breyer.* Retrieved from https://www.c-span.org/video/?286074-1/supreme-court-justice-breyer

Davis, J. H. (2017, April 10). Neil Gorsuch is sworn in as Supreme Court justice. *The New York Times.* Retrieved from https://www.nytimes.com/2017/04/10/us/politics/neil-gorsuch-supreme-court.html?_r=0

Delaney, J. (2011). *Learning legal reasoning: Briefing, analysis and theory.* Catskill, NY. Delaney Publications.

Erie Railroad Company v. Tompkins, 304 U.S. 64. (1938). Retrieved from https://supreme.justia.com/cases/federal/us/304/64/case.html

Fact sheet. (2000). *Planned Parenthood Federation of America.* New York, NY: Katharine Dexter McCormick Library. Retrieved from http://lobby.la.psu.edu/013_contraceptive_coverage/organizational_statements/Planned_Parenthood/Planned_Parenthood_The_Impact_of_Legal_Birth_Control.htm

Federal Rules of Civil Procedure. (2016). *Current rules of practice & procedure.* Retrieved from www.uscourts.gov/rules-policies/current-rules-practice-procedure

Garvin, D. A. (2003, September–October). Making the case: Professional education for the world of practice. *Harvard Magazine.* Retrieved from http://harvardmagazine.com/2003/09/making-the-case-html

Gomberg, L. J. (circa 1990). Notes and flowchart for lectures on civil procedure for Western State University class in Civil Procedure. Copies in possession of Linda J. Gomberg.

Gomberg, L. J. (2012). *The case for privacy: A history of privacy in the United States as seen through a psychological lens and defined by case law and the impact of social media* (PhD Doctoral dissertation). Fielding Graduate University, California. Retrieved from http://search.proquest.com.proxy1.library.jhu.edu/docview/921498079

Griswold v. Connecticut, 381 U.S. 479 (1965).

Hoeflich, M. H. (1989). Law, culture, and the university: An inaugural discourse. *Syracuse Law Review, 20,* 789–797.

Jarrett, L. (2017, March 16). Trump admin to appeal travel ban rulings "soon." *CNN Politics.* Retrieved from http://www.cnn.com/2017/03/15/politics/travel-ban-blocked/

Maslow, A. H. (1950). Self-actualizing people: A study of psychological health. *Personality.* pp. 11–34.

Munson, H. (2013). FAQ: Basic facts about the Bill of Rights. *Constitution Daily.* Retrieved from https://constitutioncenter.org/blog/everything-you-ever-wanted-to-know-about-the-bill-of-rights.

Newland, E. (2015). Executive orders in court. *The Yale Law Journal, 124,* 2026–2099.

Revisiting a landmark birth control ruling, 50 years later. (2015, June 7). *Newsweek.* Retrieved from http://www.newsweek.com/revisiting-landmark-birth-control-ruling-fifty-years-339559

Walsh, K. T. (2010, March 12). The 1960s: A decade of change for women. *US News and World Report.* Retrieved from https://www.usnews.com/topics/author/kenneth-t-walsh

How They Met: Behavior and the Law

OVERVIEW

In Chapter 1, the separate historical origins of the inevitable meeting of law and psychology were introduced and explored to explain how the "forensic" aspect came to be part of the world of psychology. Although forensic psychologists are trained first as psychologists, they need to have a certain depth of understanding of the law and legal systems within which they will work. Chapter 2 provided a foundation in Constitutional law and how our legal systems and all branches of our government were created and function from that base. While those first two chapters sought to provide depth, or the roots, for the topic, Part I concludes with this chapter, which addresses the origins of the breadth of the topic. This chapter not only shows how behavior and the law met and got together, but also gets specific about how the two are inextricably intertwined in the United States and how certain aspects of that intertwining became and remain forensic psychology. Two constructs in the study of law and psychology, **context** and perception, are used to illustrate just how the two disciplines work together and how they can be distinguished from each other. Context and perception in both disciplines provide meaning in and for any given situation, both in the way they overlap and in their separateness.

The two earlier chapters presented cases illustrative of particular points made in the chapters. This chapter continues that method with the case of *Elonis v. United States* (2015), not only to illustrate the main constructs under discussion, but also because the case encompasses so many psychological and legal issues. Thus, it also serves as an incentive for follow-up discussions.

This chapter also includes the first of a series of interviews with individuals who work in the field. Dr. James Earnest is employed as a forensic psychologist and shares how he achieved his employment goal and what he has been doing for the county for which he works for almost 20 years.

HOW IT WORKS

The "it" in this chapter is the breadth of forensic psychology. Psychologists and lawyers look at all situations in relation to the context. They are always aware of whose perception will be considered.

Context

Generally, context is a frame of reference; it is situational. Although many examples will be used throughout this chapter to illustrate the term and its impact in both law and psychology, one very common example might explain it best. Who among us has not participated in, watched, or listened to at least part of a "spelling bee," the contest that through the process of elimination allegedly produces the best speller among a group of usually young contestants? Frequently, after being given an unfamiliar word, a contestant will ask for the word to be used in a sentence. This will provide the context or the place that gives the word meaning and possibly help the contestant come up with the correct spelling. In reading through this chapter, that lesson might be helpful in thinking about how looking to the context of a problem (be it psychology, law, or a combination of both) often helps resolve the problem.

In Psychology

Psychology is the study of human behavior. To understand that behavior, it must be viewed situationally and environmentally (King, Viney, & Woody, 2013). Context is a term of cognitive psychology, the study of mental processes. This includes the study of memory, thought, and intelligence (King et al., 2013). Context is also a term of social psychology, as that discipline involves relationships, human interaction, and groups; the context changes accordingly (Aronson, 2012; Matsumoto, 2007). Although discussing context as a completely separate topic from perception is more difficult in psychology than it is in the law, the attempt needs to be made before bringing the two constructs together.

One of the oldest and best examples of context in regard to behavior that is not subjective and, therefore, does not merge with perception should be familiar to all: The mother admonishes her children who have been yelling from room to room in their home, or the teacher tries to get her students to raise their hands rather than shout out answers or questions while in a classroom. Their method of creating order is the same; the children are cautioned to use their "inside voices." In the playground or even the school yard, of course, the loud laughter or even shouting is acceptable. This is context. In fact, a recent observation in an outdoor strip mall serves as an even more relevant example. A somewhat oddly dressed middle-aged woman was ostentatiously parading outside various stores and restaurants with a cell phone to her ear. Passersby were avoiding her until a group of four or five preteens seemed to be in her way. The children were laughing and talking while being followed by three or four adults. The woman began shouting at the children to be quiet as she was on the phone. One of the adults laughingly said, "We are outside, and they are using their outside voices." Again, this is context.

Psychology students quickly learn that studying behavior means studying the context of that behavior. As illustrated in the preceding examples, what is standard in some situations is unacceptable in others. The diversity of our society, including our cultural influences, also reminds us of the importance of examining the context of the circumstances. Matsumoto (2007) posits that behavior comes from three sources: psychological processes or personality, basic human nature, and culture. Which of these sources is dominant in the social role of an individual at any given time is dependent upon the context (Matsumoto, 2007). As will be seen later, if culture is given the generic definition of group membership with roots in social psychology, the meaning and influence of culture on context become apparent. Myriad research articles are published every year describing the role that context plays in human behavior and how that behavior should be interpreted depending upon the context. A quick computer search for peer-reviewed publications during a 2-year span revealed over 25,000 articles based in the social sciences that were either about context or had the word in their title (Google "context in social sciences" + "peer reviewed").

For those who expect to be clinicians, the context of a therapeutic interview versus that of a forensic interview takes on much importance. The psychologist in a therapeutic interview is an advocate interviewing a client, usually the person paying the bill. The clinician's concern is how best to help that client (American Psychological Association, 2017). The context of a clinical interview is one of therapist and client. The clinician approaches the client with **empathy** and understanding, assuming that what is going to transpire is based on honesty and a desire to be helped by the clinician (Rogers, 1975). The client's presence is voluntary, and the role of the clinician is to act in the best interest of the client. The forensic interview is different; the situation and, therefore, the context are different—even though the mental health professional may actually have the same training and act as a therapist in other circumstances. When acting in a forensic capacity, the clinician is an objective party, conducting an objective investigation of the individual presented (American Psychological Association, 2013). That individual may or may not be the client, but the interview is for the purpose of some court-ordered or at least court-interested matter. The clinician in this case is advised to see the individual with a more critical eye—some might even say cynically. The situation or context is one of evaluator and examinee. The forensic psychologist might be receiving compensation from an attorney or the court. If compensation is being paid by the participant, the relationship becomes a bit more complicated, and the individual could become the client (American Psychological Association, 2013). This is not to say, however, that the psychologist does not have other fiduciary obligations when acting in a forensic setting. The possibility of conflicting dual roles can present ethical issues for the clinician. In fact, Guideline 4.02.03 of the *Specialty Guidelines for Forensic Psychology* (American Psychological Association, 2013) states in part that "Forensic practitioners are encouraged" to consider the effects therapeutic services can have "when they provide therapeutic services in forensic contexts" (p. 4). Such services can have unintended negative effects on future legal proceedings or the therapy itself according to the Specialty Guidelines (American Psychological Association, 2013).

Table 3.1 lays out the general differences regarding the two types of services.

In the Law

Age is an excellent example of understanding how context works in the law. While the eligible age for a juror is 18 years in most jurisdictions in the United States, the actual age range of jurors tends to be between 35 and 65; one study that researched juror attitudes found that the mean age of 139 jurors was 41.5 years (Lehmann & Smith, 2013). It is a well-known fact that most social science research is conducted with undergraduate college students, and since that research is usually conducted by academicians with university appointments, the participants are actually what is known as a **convenience sample**. In reviewing articles submitted for publication and/or presentation for Division 41 of the American Psychological Association, it is not unusual to read that the participants were hundreds of college students utilized for various research purposes. A couple of years ago, one submission in particular stood out: Researchers had

TABLE 3.1 Forensic Versus Clinical Interview

	Forensic Interview	Clinical Interview
GOAL/PURPOSE OF INTERVIEW	Establish relevant facts/address referral question from client. Lay foundation for expert opinion requested.	Client initiates interview, seeking relief of symptoms/ issues. Assist client in understanding problems. Help client achieve behavioral change.
MENTAL HEALTH PROFESSIONAL'S ROLE	Understand and satisfy the legal issue(s) involved. Do not come to legal conclusions. Be aware of and inform examinee that information is being prepared for and could be used by attorneys, court, or other individuals/ agencies.	Fiduciary of client who has explained limits (minor in most instances) of confidentiality and other salient issues. Satisfaction of client needs. Information used for client's benefit/ welfare unless legal mandatory reporting. Record keeping and reporting informal for client's benefit.
PSYCHOLOGIST'S ASSUMPTIONS	Do not assume, presume, or predict. Examinee's perception may be skewed/not truthful. Client may have personal/professional stake in the outcome, but is not the examinee (usually). Maintain objectivity.	Client is telling the truth as client knows it (perception). Client's distress is genuine. Client needs professional support.

(*continued*)

TABLE 3.1 Forensic Versus Clinical Interview (*continued*)

METHOD/ TECHNIQUE	Assess cognitive and other psychological processes through interview and instruments. Raise client's level to evaluator's level. Avoid suggestion, encourage detail, and record (audio/video) if possible.	Utilize theoretical orientation best suited to/for particular client/issue. Assume client's level. Use suggestion, inference, or interpretation of deeper meanings in expression. Empathy.

enrolled over 500 college students, average age 19 years, as mock jurors responding to one question about the credibility of expert testimony. Although this research obviously was time-consuming, and the authors thought they had enough responses to generalize their findings, the findings were not applicable to the situation or the context. The 500 participants with an average age of 19 years could not represent 12 actual jurors. In fact, Wiener, Krauss, and Lieberman (2011) compared responses of college students acting as mock jurors with older adults whom they called "eligible jurors" (p. 477). They concluded that although utilizing college students as mock jurors was efficient, jury studies that use only these undergraduates lack validity and generalizability (Wiener et al., 2011). In contrast, in 2017 the Harvard Kennedy School's Institute of Politics conducted a poll specifically for the purpose of finding out what young adults think about a particular topic. In this context, the 18- to 29-year olds who responded were the appropriate participants.

Of course, using the age of jurors as an example of context in law may also be viewed as an example of context in psychology. Much jury research is conducted by psychologists and, as noted earlier, submitted for publication to the American Psychological Association.

More to the point, then, context in the law can be explained by the method most law schools use to teach their students. As was explained in Chapter 2, when Christopher Columbus Langdell became Dean of Harvard Law School in 1870, he brought with him several new and innovative ideas for legal education. Among those ideas was using actual cases to teach the law students; this **casebook method** has since become the standard not only for law school teaching, but also in many business and medical schools (Garvin, 2003). This is mentioned again here because prior to the tenure of Langdell, the study of law consisted of rote learning of statutes through lecture and drills, with little or no student input (Garvin, 2003). Langdell's goal was for students to not just learn, but to understand the law through the analysis of the real issues and resolutions with which they would be dealing. What Langdell was doing, then, was putting the law in context for the students. Through the facts of a particular case, they could more readily understand and work with the issues presented and the application of the relevant laws. Again, when the problem is put into the appropriate context, it is much more easily and accurately resolved.

This legal context is demonstrated even more specifically in the **Amicus Curiae brief** submitted to the court by the American Civil Liberties Union (ACLU) and others in support of the appeal of Anthony Elonis to the United States (U.S.) Supreme Court in *Elonis v. United States*, 2015 (Brief for the American Civil Liberties Union as Amici Curiae Supporting Petitioner, *Elonis v. United States* [no. 13-983], 2014) (see the case later in this chapter). In arguing that the jury instructions were improperly submitted to the jury, the brief states, "A properly charged jury might or might not have concluded that [Mr. Elonis' postings] also constituted a threat in context" (p. 4). The brief goes on to say that the jury should have been allowed to consider "more evidence contextualizing the online comment" than was admitted (p. 27).

Perception

Perception is point of view. It is the subjective understanding of the observer. Whether it is reality, or another's reality, is not always the point. Perception is subjective.

In Psychology

By now you are probably no longer wondering why it is so difficult to separate context from perception in psychology, as no clear lines exist between the constructs. Using the earlier example of culture as one of the driving forces of behavior, the term "fraternity culture" has recently become popular when describing life among these college-based social groups (Bennett, 2014, para. 9; Matsumoto, 2007). Although by 2014 fraternity hazing had become illegal in 44 states, very few college-based fraternities observed those laws (Parks, Jones, & Hughey, 2015). Hazing is defined as "an abusive, often humiliating form of initiation into or affiliation with a group" (Hazing Law and Legal Definition, n.d., para. 1). This includes "[Any] willful action taken or situation created which recklessly or intentionally endangers the mental or physical health of another" (Hazing Law and Legal Definition, n.d., para. 2). Although the human desire to be one of a group and/or conform to the ways of that group is understood, one still cannot help but wonder why anyone would subject himself to that humiliation and sometimes even dangerous situation. Regardless, fraternities justify hazing as an initiation into a club, a rite of passage that the older members had all undergone, and state that new members consented to the process by joining the fraternities (Stolberg, 2017). The context, then, is one of group members usually living together and partying together. They call themselves brothers in this context, and this is the way they are perceived by those wanting to join. There are many cases where this context and the perception of it have resulted in negative outcomes, and a specific one that further illustrates the unique context that contributes to the perception of those involved is described in the "In the News" feature in this chapter.

Empathy is a term often used in the clinical practice of psychology. It connotes a therapist being able to step into the shoes of the client and perceive the world through the client's eyes. It is a skill learned only through training and experience, with experience being the more operative word. In 1975, Carl Rogers, who was known for his humanistic and client-centered approach to therapy, found empathy to be such an important construct that he admitted to defining and redefining it over a period of more than 20 years. He went from defining empathy as a state of perceiving "the internal frame of reference of another with accuracy" (p. 3)—a definition that he had published in 1959—to deciding empathy was a process by which one enters "the private perceptual world of the other and [becomes] thoroughly at home in it" (p. 4). While Carl Rogers' definition of the term gives credibility to the need for the therapist to understand and be able to implement empathy, the purpose of establishing how the construct of perception applies in a psychological setting and understanding the mental health professionals' display of empathy during the therapeutic relationship relates to psychology's understanding of perception.

In the Law

In law, psychology, and the events of everyday life, perception is the point of view of the individuals involved. Since perception is subjective, it may seem strange and even contradictory that the law attributes certain aspects of perception to the individuals who come into court, and the perception attributed is dependent upon the role of the individual. An almost one-century-old torts case illustrates this construct. The facts were a simple and familiar landlord/tenant dispute. The tenant did not pay rent and was moving out, taking her belongings with her. The landlord pointed a gun at the tenant and her movers, threatening to shoot if the tenant did not leave her belongings on the premises as payment for the overdue rent. The landlord sued the tenant for the overdue rent, and the tenant sued the landlord for civil assault.[1] Assault is and was defined as the intentional placing of another in fear of imminent harm; the tenant claimed having a gun pointed at her put her in fear of imminent harm. The landlord defended herself on the grounds that the gun was unloaded, so she did not have the means to harm the plaintiff tenant. The plaintiff won, based on the facts of the case and the applicable law. The court stated the tort of assault existed when the plaintiff perceived he or she was in danger of imminent harm (*Allen v. Hannaford*, 1926). The knowledge on the part of the defendant that she could not have harmed the tenant with the unloaded gun did not negate the intentional pointing of the gun and the apprehension of the plaintiff.

SPOTLIGHT ON CASES

Some Background

Just as *Allen v. Hannaford* (1926) seems to have set the standard for establishing civil intent (dependent on context of the situation and perception of the plaintiff), decades later a U.S. Supreme Court case, *Elonis v. United States* (2015), not only illustrates that same construct but goes even further to illustrate what is necessary to establish criminal intent. In criminal law, the perception or intent of the defendant is the standard. In fact, in his dissent, Justice Clarence Thomas stated the court had agreed to hear the case so the court could finally resolve the question of the requisite mental state of the defendant needed to convict under the criminal statute.[2]

Aside from illustrating some of the overlapping psychological and legal constructs of this chapter, this case is a product of its time. While the broad issues presented and the ruling by the Supreme Court both draw on precedent and will be applied in the future, the facts of *Elonis v. United States* (2015) could have arisen only in this modern context. A further statement about the importance of context comes from the case itself: In his dissent, Justice Samuel Alito referred to the difference in interpretation of language depending on the context. If the language was that of song lyrics, it could and should be interpreted quite differently than if it was merely a fear-inducing statement on social media (*Elonis v. United States*, 2015).

Elonis v. United States (2015)

Facts: After 7 years of marriage, Anthony Elonis' wife took their two children and left him. He had been an active Facebook user, but after his wife left, he began using a pseudonym and posted threatening-sounding language on his Facebook page. His wife stated she was frightened and was able to get a restraining order against him. His behavior at work became unprofessional and inappropriate, causing his boss to fire him. Coworkers claimed to be uncomfortable and afraid to be around him. At one point, Elonis posted a photo on Facebook depicting him holding a knife to the throat of a female coworker with a caption that read, "I wish." His posts were filled with swear words and threats, often in the form of rap-style lyrics, about shooting up kindergarten classes, dismembering his estranged wife, blowing up the police, and harming his former employer. Intermixed in his posts were various types of disclaimers categorizing the posts as potential rap lyrics. Because of the specificity of his threatening words, posted picture, and other odd behaviors, Elonis' former employer, who had access to his Facebook account, went to the local police and the Federal Bureau of Investigation (FBI) with the information.

The FBI investigation provided enough evidence to arrest Elonis.

Procedural History: Elonis was then tried and convicted in federal district court in Philadelphia for violating a federal criminal law making it illegal to transmit a threat to kidnap or injure another person through interstate commerce. By posting the threats on Facebook, Elonis was deemed to have been transmitting through interstate commerce. Punishment under the statute was a fine, up to 5 years in prison, or both (Crimes & Criminal Procedure 18 U.S.C § 875(c), 1940). His conviction was affirmed by the Third Circuit Court of Appeals, and by the time his appeal was heard by the U.S. Supreme Court, Anthony Elonis had been in prison for 3 years.

Issue: Over Mr. Elonis' objection, the jury had been instructed that the defendant was guilty if a reasonable person would have understood his words to be threats. Mr. Elonis had asked that the jury be instructed to base its decision on Mr. Elonis' intent, meaning whether he actually intended to harm the individuals he named in his posts.

As has been stated, the U.S. Supreme Court does not have to hear most of the cases that are brought to it and selects only a very few cases to consider each term. Here, although the court used language asking if Mr. Elonis' postings were true threats, the basic question of the decision that had to be made was if it was the mental state of the defendant in regard to his postings that should be under consideration—that is, whether he actually intended to harm anyone with his seemingly threatening words, or whether the consideration by the jury should have been if others were truly frightened or put in fear of imminent harm by his words.

Holding: According to the lower courts, all that was required was the perception of a reasonable person as to whether the defendant's words would cause that fear in others. According to the U.S. Supreme Court, however, the standard was quite different. Although the majority opinion did not use the exact language, it did follow previously established interpretations of perception from earlier cases. The majority opinion stated that Mr. Elonis had been convicted of violating a criminal statute, and the criminal process in such a case requires the defendant to have the intent, the *mens rea*, or guilty mind to do harm. This was not what the jury heard in its instruction.

Judgment: Seven of the nine U.S. Supreme Court justices agreed that the appeals court should be reversed and the case remanded.

Elonis Epilogue

However, there is a twist. While this case works well to illustrate both context and perception for these legal purposes, upon remand, the Third Circuit Court of Appeals called the jury instruction "harmless error" and maintained that the jury would have convicted Anthony Elonis even if it had been correctly instructed. In reiterating the facts of the case, the Third Circuit came to the conclusion that since the Supreme Court did not give a specific test for determining the intent of the defendant, the evidence clearly showed that Elonis knew that his words would cause fear and that his purpose was to threaten the parties to whom the threats were made (*United States v. Elonis*, 2016).

FOCUS ON CAREERS

James Earnest, PhD, ABPP, understands context and perception, including the importance of both and the distinction between the two, in the legal and psychological environs within which he works. He spends his work days divided

(*continued*)

(continued)

between evaluating patients in psychiatric hospitals and reporting his findings in court. He needs to be mindful of the perceptions of the patients, attorneys, and judges who make the final decisions when he evaluates and makes his recommendations regarding the fitness of those patients for release (CA W & I Code §5150 et seq.)

When Dr. Earnest earned his PhD in clinical psychology, he opened a private practice servicing outpatient clients but heavily populated with an inpatient caseload as well. He expected this to be his lifelong career. Within a few years, however, managed healthcare became the primary provider of health services, private practice was disappearing, and fewer mental health clients were occupying inpatient hospital beds. Dr. Earnest saw the changes and purposely "retooled" himself to be in a position to be hired by the county as a forensic psychologist. He reconnected with a former mentor, who helped him gain the experience and further education necessary put himself in a position to be hired by the county as a full-time employee. He also achieved membership in the American Board of Professional Psychology (ABPP), an extremely selective organization that restricts its membership to only 4,000 highly qualified practicing psychologists (ABPP, n.d.).

After a decade of gaining experience, continuing his education, and conducting over 200 child custody evaluations as a court-appointed psychologist, Dr. Earnest was hired as a forensic psychologist by the county's healthcare agency in Adult and Older Adult Behavioral Health Services. Almost 20 years later, he remains one of four county forensic psychologists referred to as "Public Guardians." His position is one that takes his expertise to conduct evaluations and testify in civil court.

Under California's Lanterman–Petris–Short Act (1967/2016), Dr. Earnest evaluates and testifies as to the competency

(continued)

(*continued*)

of individuals involuntarily committed as "gravely disabled" (CA Welfare & Institutions Code §5150). In preparation for his testimony, Dr. Earnest reviews the patient's history and mental health record, goes to the inpatient facility, and interviews the patient, who in compliance with the statute has been committed for 72 hours or 14 days, depending upon the circumstances of the individual case. As an experienced forensic psychologist, Dr. Earnest knows what questions to ask and what kinds of responses the court wants to hear to do its own evaluation and make a decision regarding the mental health of the patient. Sometimes the patients acknowledge they are incapable of living on their own, in which case Dr. Earnest's report ends the proceeding for the time being. However, the majority of cases, which might include individuals with schizophrenia, suicidal individuals, substance abusers, and/ or those whose behavior is considered potentially dangerous to others, end up being set for a hearing. Currently, in fact, Dr. Earnest has at least one scheduled jury trial.

In the past, Jim Earnest, PhD, was referred to as an "expert forensic psychologist" when he evaluated the defendant and testified during the trial of a woman who was contesting and later appealed the appointment of a conservator (*Conservatorship of the Person and Estate of Shirley T.*, 2014). Dr. Earnest testified that after evaluating Shirley, he diagnosed her as schizophrenic and "gravely disabled" under the provisions of the statute, thereby requiring the conservatorship (CA Welfare & Institutions Code §5150). His evaluation and recommendation were based on interviewing Shirley at the facility, speaking with the facility's professional staff, reviewing the patient's medical and psychiatric records, and reviewing the previously appointed guardian's investigative report (*Conservatorship of the Person and Estate of Shirley T.*, 2014). The appeals court affirmed the earlier decision after quoting Dr. Earnest's testimony. While it is

(*continued*)

(*continued*)

> probably unusual for a conservatorship case to be appealed, having the record of the actual work of a forensic psychologist at work in the courts provides insight into the career Dr. Earnest has chosen.
>
> Dr. Earnest also teaches master's and doctoral forensic psychology students. They know how fortunate they are that he gives them the opportunity to see the daily life of a forensic psychologist when he invites them to court during one of his "testifying" days.

IN THE NEWS

In February 2017, a 19-year-old man pledging a fraternity at Pennsylvania State University died of injuries suffered as a result of an alcohol-abusive hazing night. On autopsy, his blood alcohol level was measured at a dangerous 0.40, and videotapes of the previous night revealed he had fallen and suffered injuries throughout the night (Stolberg, 2017). Eighteen fraternity members were indicted by a grand jury, all on misdemeanor counts and a few on one or two felony counts as well (Miller, 2017). Although fraternity and sorority hazing has been outlawed on almost all college campuses, enforcement was obviously lax on the Penn State campus in early 2017. Unfortunately, this incident is not unusual. As stated earlier in the chapter, much of this behavior has been attributed to the "fraternity culture" that seems to allow those participating to perceive these events within the context of that culture, so that it becomes a new definition of normal.

SUMMARY

This final chapter of Part I brought together two major constructs in the law and psychology to illustrate how the two disciplines are intertwined and yet need to be distinguished. The constructs, context and perception were not only illustrated in regard to how they operate in psychology and the law, but specific cases further illustrated the place of the terms in the discipline.

These constructs were also relevant to the work of the forensic psychologist, Dr. James Earnest, who was fittingly profiled for this particular chapter. Since he spends his professional time in the courts and in psychiatric hospitals, the importance of context to the work he does is easily identified.

Just as profiling a working forensic psychologist makes the constructs presented easier to understand, finding and providing real-life stories about the somewhat abstract concepts creates a concrete frame of reference. The issue of fraternity hazing has been in the news of late, and was included to make the point of the relevance of the topic and to demonstrate how context can define culture.

DISCUSSION QUESTIONS

1. Below are excerpts from the "rap lyrics" that Anthony Elonis posted on Facebook. From reading the brief in this chapter, including the facts of the case and these few examples, what do you think was Mr. Elonis' intent?

   Did you know that it's illegal for me to say I want to kill my wife? . . . It's one of the only sentences that I'm not allowed to say. . . . Now it was okay for me to say it right then because I was just telling you that it's illegal for me to say I want to kill my wife. . . . . . . it's very illegal to say I really, really think someone out there should kill my wife. . . . But not illegal to say with a mortar launcher. Because that's its own sentence. . . . (*Elonis v. United States*, 2015, p. 3).

   You know your s***'s ridiculous when you have the FBI knockin' at yo' door
   Little Agent lady stood so close
   Took all the strength I had not to turn the b**** ghost
   Pull my knife, flick my wrist, and slit her throat

Leave her bleedin' from her jugular in the arms of her
  partner [laughter]
So the next time you knock, you best be serving a warrant
And bring yo' SWAT and an explosives expert while you're at it
Cause little did y'all know, I was strapped wit' a bomb
Why do you think it took me so long to get dressed with
  no shoes on?
I was jus' waitin' for y'all to handcuff me and pat me down
Touch the detonator in my pocket and we're all goin'
  [BOOM!] Are all the pieces comin' together? S***, I'm
  just a crazy sociopath (*Elonis v. United States*, 2015, p. 5).

2. Using a broad definition of culture as used in the chapter, individuals can and do belong to many cultures simultaneously. Discuss the various cultures or groups to which you belong and how and if your behavior might change according to the group you are in.

NOTES

1. There is a criminal counterpart to assault, but it is most often merged into the more serious crime of battery. Florida's definition of battery, the intentional unconsented touching or striking of another, is indicative of the common law and other state definitions (Chapter 784, 2017).
2. The statute under which Mr. Elonis was convicted reads in part: "Whoever transmits in interstate or foreign commerce any communication containing any threat to kidnap any person or any threat to injure the person of another, shall be fined under this title or imprisoned not more than 5 years, or both" (Crimes & Criminal Procedure 18 U.S.C. § 875 (c), 1940).

REFERENCES

Allen v. Hannaford, 138 Wash. 423 (1926).

American Board of Professional Psychology (ABPP). (n.d.). Retrieved from https://www.abpp.org/i4a/pages/index.cfm?pageid=3341

American Psychological Association. (2013). Specialty guidelines for forensic psychology. *American Psychologist, 68*(1), 7–19. doi:10.1037/a0029889

American Psychological Association. (2017). *Ethical principles of psychologists and code of conduct*. Washington, DC: Author. Retrieved from http://www.apa.org/ethics/code/ethics-code-2017.pdf

Aronson, E. (2012). *The social animal* (11th ed.). New York, NY: Worth.

Bennett, J. (2014, December). The problem with frats isn't just rape. It's power. *Time*. Retrieved from http://time.com/3616158/fraternity-rape-uva-rolling-stone-sexual-assault/

Brief for the American Civil Liberties Union as Amici Curiae Supporting Petitioner, *Elonis v. United States* (no. 13-983). (2014). Retrieved from https://www.aclu.org/legal-document/elonis-v-united-states-amicus-brief

Chapter 784: Assault; Battery; Culpable Negligence. 2017 Florida Statutes. § 784.03 (2017).

Conservatorship of the Person and Estate of Shirley T. No.G050372 (4th Appellate Dist. Div. 3 2014).

Crimes & Criminal Procedure 18 U.S.C. § 875 (1940). Retrieved from https://www.gpo.gov/fdsys/pkg/USCODE-2011-title18/pdf/USCODE-2011-title18-partI-chap41-sec875.pdf

Elonis v. United States, 135 S. Ct. 2001 (2015).

Garvin, D. A. (2003, September–October). Making the case. *Harvard Magazine*, *106*(1). Retrieved from harvardmag.com/pdf/2003/09-pdfs/0903-56.pdf

Harvard Institute of Politics. (2017, April 25). As first 100 days nears, President Trump approval rating at 32% with young Americans, Harvard poll finds. Retrieved from http://iop.harvard.edu/youth-poll/harvard-iop-spring-17-poll

Hazing Law and Legal Definition (n.d.). Legal definitions. *USLegal*. Retrieved from https://definitions.uslegal.com/h/hazing/

King, B. D., Viney, W., & Woody, W. D. (2013). *A history of psychology ideas and context*. New York, NY: Taylor & Francis.

Lanterman–Petris–Short Act, CA Welfare & Institutions Code §§ 5000-8000 (1967/2016).

Lehmann, J. K., & Smith, J. B. (2013). *A multidimensional examination of jury composition, trial outcomes, and attorney preferences* (NBER Working Paper 17450). Retrieved from http://www.uh.edu/~jlehman2/papers/lehmann_smith_jurycomposition.pdf

Matsumoto, D. (2007). Culture, context, and behavior. *Journal of Personality*, *75*(6), 1285–1319.

Miller, S. P. (2017, May 5). Beta Theta Pi fraternity and 18 brothers charged in death of Timothy Piazza; 8 facing manslaughter charges. County of Centre, Commonwealth of Pennsylvania, Office of the District Attorney. Retrieved from https://www.scribd.com/document/347431625/Notice-11-FINAL-Charges-and-Presentment#from_embed

Parks, G. S., Jones, S. E., & Hughey, M. W. (2015). *Hazing as a crime: An empirical analysis of criminological antecedents* (Wake Forest University Legal Studies Paper No. 2405079). Retrieved from https://papers.ssrn.com/sol3/papers.cfm?abstract_id=2405079

Rogers, C. R. (1975). Empathic: An unappreciated way of being. *Counseling Psychologist, 5*(2), 2–10.

Stolberg, S. G. (2017, May 5). 18 Penn State students charged in fraternity death. *New York Times.* Retrieved from https://www.nytimes.com/2017/05/05/us/penn-state-fraternity-death-timothy-piazza.html

United States v. Elonis No. 12.3798 (3rd Cir. Oct. 28. 2016)

Wiener, R. L., Krauss, D. A., & Lieberman, J. D. (2011). Mock jury research: Where do we go from here? *Behavioral Sciences and the Law, 29,* 457–479. doi:10.1002/bsl.989

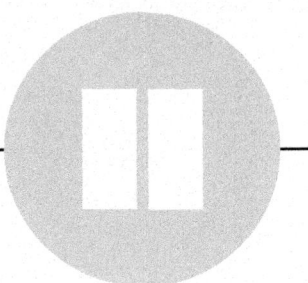

Forensic Psychologists in the Courts

Criminal Matters: Ethics, Types of Crimes, and Criminal Cases

OVERVIEW

This chapter highlights the various roles that a forensic psychologist might play during the course and within the context of a **criminal trial**. Although state laws differ regarding specific wording of **statutes** and in sentencing requirements, generally all criminal trials follow the same basic format. From the inception of the process, forensic psychologists may be called upon to evaluate not only **competency** to proceed at various points, but also **malingering** and **mitigating circumstances**. In states that allow such pleas, these psychologists evaluate for and testify about such defenses as **not guilty by reason of insanity** (NGRI) and **guilty but mentally incompetent** (GBMI). Some are trained to be **sex offender risk evaluators** as well as evaluators for various other types of criminal risk assessments, such as the likelihood of **recidivism** and **domestic violence**. In some cases, forensic psychologists are employed by law enforcement to evaluate capacity and to aid in questioning suspects. The forensic psychologist may have a role before, during, and even after the criminal trial is over. As was seen in Chapter 3, providing that context should clarify those roles.

This chapter also presents an opportunity to discuss the ethics of expert testimony, interrogation of suspects, and the psycholegal issues presented in criminal matters. Some of these issues will be illustrated by using cases made popular by television and social media. The cases highlighting these points are the murder trials of **Jody Arias** in Arizona and **Brendan Dassey**, who was living in Wisconsin but had his case deliberated in federal court.

Cases that have become precedent setting due to the input of psychologists and others are explained, along with cases that present new issues and crimes for the criminal justice system—for example, the finding(s) of criminal grounds for prosecuting defendants who could not be shown to have had the requisite criminal intent to take the life of another, yet allegedly due to their behavior, a death resulted (Berman, 2017b). The trial of Michelle Carter and similar cases before hers would likely not have occurred without the development of social media. However, although she was nowhere near where the death actually took place, Carter was convicted of being instrumental in the death of a friend who committed suicide. Her story is told in the "In the News" feature.

This chapter also features profiles of two forensic psychologists. Although both work in the criminal justice system, their roles are quite different, and each has a position integral to the system, specialized, and within the career path that many future forensic psychologists hope to follow. Interviews with Drs. Adam Yerke and Trisha Elloyan provide insight into the professional lives of a sex offender evaluator and a prison psychologist, respectively.

HOW IT WORKS

In General

For the most part, criminal behavior legally requires two conditions: mens rea (the guilty mind) and actus reus (the guilty act) on the part of the defendant (Berman, 2017b). Without a confession, it is the prosecution's responsibility to prove both **beyond a reasonable doubt** to secure a **conviction**. This is the **burden of proof** in a criminal proceeding. On the other side, although the policy of our legal system is that all defendants are innocent until proven guilty, the defense has the responsibility to counter the prosecution's arguments and at the very least plant that reasonable doubt in the minds of the triers of fact (*Coffin v. United States*, 1895). During the course of a criminal prosecution, both sides have many opportunities to procure the services of a forensic psychologist. Because the defense is continually working to secure the release of the defendant, following the course of those opportunities throughout the trial will explain the key points for both sides. When appropriate, certain relevant and/or precedent-setting cases are referenced as well.

The Case Begins

When a crime has occurred, law enforcement investigates to find the perpetrator or perpetrators. To put the problem into context, assume a criminal homicide, the killing of one human being by another without excuse or justification, has occurred (Homicide definition, 2013). Further assume that the dead body is nude and is rife with both stab and gunshot wounds, allowing law enforcement to immediately determine the case at hand is a criminal act (Berman, 2017a).[1] For further context, when applicable, much of what follows (as the facts of the homicide in our example case) will be taken from the reported trial of Jody Arias, who was accused and eventually convicted of murdering Travis Alexander in his shower in Arizona in 2008 (McLaughlin, 2013). Jody Arias's trial was particularly interesting in terms of the use of expert testimony from purported forensic mental health professionals.

The Trial

While the focus of the discussion here is the actual trial process, the case begins when the crime is discovered. Although the forensic psychologist may not become involved until the trial has begun or even until there is an appeal of the trial verdict, the services to be provided might involve expert opinions/evaluations from any prior time (Figure 4.1).

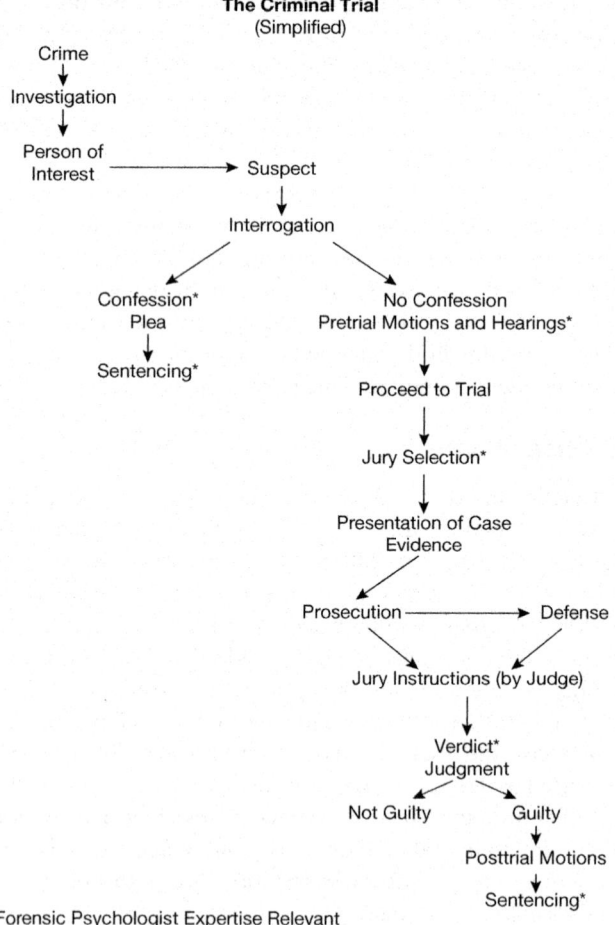

The Criminal Trial
(Simplified)

Crime
↓
Investigation
↓
Person of Interest → Suspect
↓
Interrogation

Confession*
Plea
↓
Sentencing*

No Confession
Pretrial Motions and Hearings*
↓
Proceed to Trial
↓
Jury Selection*
↓
Presentation of Case Evidence

Prosecution → Defense

Jury Instructions (by Judge)
↓
Verdict*
Judgment

Not Guilty   Guilty
↓
Posttrial Motions
↓
Sentencing*

*Forensic Psychologist Expertise Relevant

FIGURE 4.1 The criminal trial (simplified).

Pretrial and Pretrial Motions

In both criminal and civil trials, the defense attorney's main job is to get the case over and done with at the earliest possible time. Therefore, the concentration is on the probable course of a criminal trial, but much of what follows might also be applicable to a civil proceeding. From the defendant's perspective, an early move to dismiss the case is at the least cost saving, and in criminal matters it could be life-saving. Prior to the trial, the criminal defense attorney, as the defendant's advocate, will use whatever legal and ethical means are available to end the process (Rangel, 2015). While numerous motions and methods can be employed by the attorney prior to the beginning of a trial on the merits of the evidence, when circumstances permit, two stand out as viable reasons for requesting a forensic evaluation be conducted.

Confessions

Criminal trials usually consist of at least two separate stages: the determination of guilt, and, if there is a guilty verdict, the sentencing stage. If, however, there has been an undisputed, voluntary, and knowing confession, there is no need for a trial to determine guilt. The motivation behind these pleas might vary from defendant to defendant, but they are often the result of **plea bargains** with the prosecution in states where such arrangments are allowed (Berman, 2017b).[2] Even if the confession is undisputed, in accepting the guilty plea, the judge will confirm that the defendant did understand the consequences of such an action (Flores, 2014). In 2011, a man named Scott Dekraai went to a local beauty salon, where his estranged wife worked, and killed her and seven other people in the worst shooting that Orange County, California, had ever endured. He was quickly arrested and said to have confessed, but it was not until 2014 that Dekraai went before a judge with his attorney and publicly declared his guilt, after which the judge explained to him that he had just become a convicted murderer (Flores, 2014). Since there was no plea bargain in this case, and the only statement about his motivation for confessing was that it was the "right thing to do," Dekraai's sentence could be either life in prison without the possibility of parole or the death penalty (Flores, 2014, para. 6; Replogle, 2017).[3]

Forensic psychology students learn as early as their initial introductory course that confessions can represent the first point of need for the services of a forensic psychologist.[4] In 1966, the **United States (U.S.) Supreme Court** heard the case of *Miranda v. Arizona*. In fact, the cases of four defendants from four different jurisdictions (three states and a federal court) had been consolidated for Supreme Court review. The four defendants, who had been arrested for a variety of unrelated felonies, had signed confessions detailing the crimes for which they had been arrested. Each of the defendants had attempted to have the confession excluded at trial based on violations of their constitutional rights in obtaining those confessions (*Miranda v. Arizona*, 1966). Among them, the defendants had been interrogated for up to 14 hours, deprived of food and water, lied to, not given the opportunity to read the written confession, and not given an explanation as to what they were signing. The question of guilt or innocence was not in front of the U.S. Supreme Court; the only question was whether the various law enforcement agencies had complied with the requirements of the **Fifth, Sixth**, and **Fourteenth Amendments** to the United States (U.S.) Constitution. The Fifth and Sixth Amendments apply to the federal government (and only one defendant was convicted under federal law), while the Fourteenth Amendment (1868) applies the rights enumerated in those amendments to state governments. The Fourteenth Amendment guarantees each citizen due process of law before being denied "life, liberty, or property" (§ 1). Therefore, if a defendant was not given the opportunity to not incriminate himself (Fifth Amendment), told why he was being arrested, or told that he had a right to an attorney (Sixth Amendment) (among other things), then he had not received due process of law as guaranteed by the Fifth and Fourteenth Amendments to the U.S. Constitution. When writing for the majority, Chief Justic Warren stated that the decision in this case did not establish new rights for criminal defendants; it merely enforced those that already existed (*Miranda v. Arizona*, 1966).

It must be kept in mind that this issue arises only in certain situations; namely, there had to have been a **confession** given during a **custodial** time. The first question that arises, especially when there is a challenge, is whether the defendant was truly in a custodial situation. If the defendant was in law enforcement custody and provided a confession, the constitutional rights iterated in *Miranda v. Arizona* (1966) had to have been read, explained, and translated if the defendant's first language is not English. Thus, if the *Miranda* warning was not read or was defective in some way prior to the confession, the first argument by the prosecution is that the confession was provided prior to the defendant being in police custody.

Those of us who watch television police shows and/or listen to news crime reports have become used to hearing that someone is a **person of interest** in a criminal matter (Chen, 2009). This has become law enforcement's way of arguing that the individual was not in custody at the time of confessing. When law enforcement acknowledges the custodial condition, the individual becomes the **suspect**, and what is now commonly referred to as the "*Miranda* warning" must be read to and understood by the individual in custody prior to any potentially incriminating statements being admissible or enforceable.

At each of the trials in what later became *Miranda v. Arizona*, the defendant was convicted of the crimes with which he had been charged. On appeal, all arguments were that the reason each defendant had been convicted was due to the wrongful admission of the unconstitutionally obtained confessions. The U.S. Supreme Court does not retry cases, and looked only to the possible constitutional violations raised by the attorneys. Included among these four cases, in fact, was one state court case that was being appealed by the state, which had lost upon the defendant's state appeal (*Miranda v. Arizona*, 1966). It is because of the decision in this case that, over 50 years later, all law enforcement officers are required to read at least four specific constitutional rights that had been violated in *Miranda v. Arizona* to all suspects in custody prior to embarking on any questioning.[5]

However, the mere reading of the rights is not always sufficient to assure the accused understands those rights (Rogers et al., 2010). Further, although there are certain basic statements that need to be made, different local jurisdictions have different scripts. Social science and legal researchers have spent decades attempting to determine just how much those warnings are understood by various groups of arrestees. If these individuals are read their rights and choose to talk to law enforcement, they are said to have **waived** their rights. This can be accomplished verbally or in writing. Rogers and colleagues (2010) looked at groups of pretrial defendants who had waived their *Miranda* rights and compared their understanding with that of college students (assuming the college students were better educated and less stressed). They found that not only were there widespread misconceptions about the meaning of some of the warnings, but those misconceptions were not significantly different in number or type between the defendants and the college students.

Grisso (1980) has researched and written extensively since the 1970s about *Miranda* rights comprehension and concluded that younger juveniles generally do not comprehend the *Miranda* rights or the consequences of waiving them. He further concluded that older teenagers (16 or older) have as much understanding as adults and maintained that was a very low standard. While his focus is on juveniles and their capacity, Grisso developed a set of instruments that has been refined at least twice over the decades and is meant to be used by forensic mental health professionals to test both juvenile and adult comprehension of the *Miranda* rights (Frumkin, Lally, & Sexton, 2012; Goldstein, Zelle, & Grisso, 2012). He even added a fifth warning to the list: The suspect is told he or she has the right to invoke those stated constitutional rights at any time (Frumkin et al., 2012). These and other instruments have been widely studied by forensic psychologists attempting to assess capacity to waive *Miranda* rights (Frumkin et al., 2012; Grisso, 1980). The standard for assessing capacity is that the defendant waived his or her rights knowingly, intelligently, and voluntarily (Blackwood, Rogers, Steadham, & Fiduccia, 2015; *Miranda v. Arizona*, 1966). The general consensus seems to be that although these instruments are helpful and provide usable results, to establish whether actual capacity exists, defendants need to complete cognitive testing, records need to be reviewed, and interviews need to be conducted. The professional who is trained to assess that capacity is the forensic psychologist, and given the right circumstances in a criminal trial, the defense attorney might want to call on one of them (Blackwood et al., 2015; Frumkin et al., 2012; Rogers et al., 2010).

No discussion of *Miranda* warnings or the issue of custodial interrogations would be complete without mentioning the case of Brendan Dassey (Demos & Ricciara, 2015). In 2015, Netflix aired a 10-part series titled *Making of a Murderer*, which tracked the saga of Steven Avery and his nephew Brendan Dassey. In 2007, the pair were convicted of killing Teresa Halbach in 2005. Avery has maintained his innocence, and the depiction of the events of his arrest, trial, and subsequent conviction for the murder of a young woman has been both lauded and criticized for its bias in Avery's favor (Thompson & Dirr, 2017). However, more relevant is that the series also brought to light the videotaped interrogation of Dassey, an allegedly cognitively challenged teenager who was interviewed by the police without the presence of his attorney (Demos & Ricciara, 2015). During the course of the interview, Dassey confessed in great detail to his role in killing the young woman. While he later tried unsuccessfully to recant the confession, at the time he incriminated not only himself, but also his uncle (Demos & Ricciara, 2015).

Much has been written about the psychology of this case, with psychologists blogging, guessing, and second guessing the decisions made (see, for example, Louszko, Torres, Effron, & Newman, 2016; Shaw, 2016; Singal, 2016). In fact, forensic psychologists were actually involved in the Dassey case. At least one forensic psychological evaluation, available online, was entered into evidence at Dassey's trial (Gordon, 2006). The report is addressed to the second of Dassey's attorneys, Mark Fremgen, who was certain that the teenager falsely confessed. Interestingly, although video of Dassey and the many psychologists and other professionals depicts a cognitively challenged young man who was always in special education classes, the forensic psychologist who evaluated him through interviews and psychological and cognitive testing found that, although he had "somewhat limited intellectual functioning," the test results showed him to be "within the 'low average' range of intelligence" or on only the "upper end of the 'borderline' range of intelligence" (Gordon, 2006, pp. 2, 3). In 2017, the Seventh Circuit Court of Appeals overturned Dassey's conviction based on evidence that his confession was not voluntary (Thompson & Dirr, 2017). The federal district court has the option of retrying him without the admission of the confession.

Not Guilty by Reason of Insanity

As discussed in Chapter 1, the legal definition of insanity has little resemblance to any psychological description. Therefore, the mental health professionals who present their evaluation findings need the specialized training that forensic psychologists acquire. The plea of Not Guilty By Reason of Insanity (NGRI) relates back to the time of commission of the crime. The defendant is admitting he or she committed the act (actus reus) but maintains the requisite intent (mens rea) was not present. As also discussed in Chapter 1, depending upon the jurisdiction, the plea might be that the defendant did not know right from wrong at the time, had an irresistible impulse, or did not understand the nature of the act (Allen, 1962; Bousfield & Merrett, 1843; Lilienfeld & Arkowitz, 2011).

The NGRI plea is not recognized in every state and is not uniformly defined among the states that do recognize it, but is a pretrial issue usually raised at the defendant's **arraignment** or a pretrial hearing. Among the vast majority of states that do recognize the plea, there is no consistency as to whom has the burden of proof and what that burden is in pleading NGRI (Burden of Proof, 2017). Some states maintain the burden is on the prosecution to prove the defendant sane beyond a reasonable doubt, while others place the burden on the defendant to prove insanity by clear and convincing evidence or even a preponderance of the evidence (Burden of Proof, 2017; California Evidence Code § 522, 2015).

Along with various other motions, pleas are entered during the pretrial phase to help frame the issues for trial. Although the process may vary somewhat from state to state and in federal court, the procedure in California serves to illustrate the general chain of events when a NGRI plea has been entered (Crimes & Punishments, 2016; Pleadings & Proceedings before Trial, 2016). In California, the defendant is allowed to enter two pleas if one is NGRI (Crimes & Punishments, 2016).[6] If this is the case, the trial on the merits ensues. If the defendant is **acquitted**, the case ends. If the defendant is guilty, the insanity phase begins with the same or a different jury as the trier of fact and the NGRI plea as an **affirmative defense** (Fry, 2017; Pleadings & Proceedings before Trial, 2016). If, however, the defendant has entered only a NGRI plea, the sole issue for jury consideration is the defendant's legally defined insanity at the time of the crime. If the jury finds the defendant was insane at the time of the crime and there is no finding of recovered sanity, the judge will order the defendant to an appropriate facility. If the jury finds the defendant was sane, the trial date will be set (Pleadings & Proceedings before Trial, 2016).

Jury Selection

After all the pretrial motions and other issues have been resolved, and the judge has determined that the defendant will go to trial. The next step is jury selection. Eligible potential jurors are summoned, usually through voting or drivers' license records, in large groups called panels. From those panels, juries are questioned through a process called **voir dire** and can be accepted or dismissed by either side or (very rarely) the judge. Each side has a certain number of preemptory challenges, challenges without objective cause, and unlimited challenges for cause.

In most states, criminal juries are made up of 12 individuals and alternates. There is no constitutional requirement that a jury be composed of 12 individuals, however, and at least one state, Florida, allows for six-person juries in criminal cases unless the death penalty is a possibility (*Williams v. Florida*, 1970). Regardless of the number of jurors, all guilty verdicts must be unanimous and beyond a reasonable doubt. Forensic psychologists may be asked to consult at least two times during this process: Jury consultants often work with the attorneys from prior to jury selection through the verdict, and in certain instances, attorneys may call on forensic psychologists to help monitor the jury selection process of the other side.

General Consulting

The popularity of a new television series seems to have created a plethora of interest in jury consulting as a career (Tedder-King & Marinakis, 2016). *Bull* features a jury consulting firm owned and operated by Dr. Jason Bull (Attanasio & McGraw, 2016). At the beginning of each episode, the narration makes very clear that he is not an attorney; instead, his job is to assist the party and attorney with jury selection, help in witness preparation, and even counsel the attorney in many instances. Dr. Bull uses modern technology to create focus groups and mock juries as well as relying on his expertise and that of his assistants (Attanasio & McGraw, 2016).

While the series is certainly entertaining, the use of technology, the creation of mirror jurors, and the ability to predict how jurors will vote are highly exaggerated (Tedder-King & Marinakis, 2016). Jury consultants do have social media at their disposal and use it to find out more about potential jurors; they do form mirror juries and poll focus groups. Nevertheless, they are not mind readers and cannot make predictions with anywhere near the 100% accuracy Dr. Bull seems to enjoy (Gomez, 2016; Tedder-King & Marinakis, 2016). Jury consultants are, for the most part, trained in the study of human behavior, and they are experts in devising a psychological strategy that involves all the parties and may serve to bring the case together (Gomez, 2016). While Dr. Bull is often seen upstaging the attorney and sometimes using questionable ethics, jury consultants clearly understand the finders of fact are the members of the jury, and they strive to work alongside the attorney and strictly within the ethical codes of both of their professions (American Psychological Association, 2013; Gomez, 2016; Tedder-King & Marinakis, 2016).

Batson–Wheeler Motion

If the more common reason for hiring jury consultants is to gain a better understanding of the psychology of the jury and the jurors' relationship to the parties, a more specific and legally based reason can often be to object to the motivation of the other side in making its challenges to potential jurors. During jury selection, the attorneys are most likely looking for opposite types of individuals, the ones who will be more sympathetic to their case. Jury consultants on both sides can advise about desirable age, gender, and social and economic status of the jurors (Lehmann & Smith, 2013). They read or engage in jury research and are prepared to evaluate which groups are more likely to convict or acquit in a given situation (Lehmann & Smith, 2013). However, when one side or the other suspects potential jurors are being stricken due to a racial bias, the law provides a remedy. In *People v. Wheeler* (1978) the California Supreme Court was tasked to review the jury selection in Wheeler's murder trial. Wheeler was black. The prosecutor used all of his preemptory challenges to excuse all black potential jurors, and the jury and two alternates were all white. This, argued the defense counsel, violates the Sixth Amendment's guarantee of a jury of one's peers, and the California court agreed (*People v. Wheeler*, 1978). In writing for the majority, Judge Mosk repeatedly made the point that juries are supposed to represent a cross-section of the community, and since many potential jurors were black, Wheeler's jury could not have represented a cross-section. *Batson v. Kentucky* (1986) raised a similar issue, but this time the case went to the U.S. Supreme Court. Only four black individuals had been called in for jury duty, but all four were quickly dismissed through preemptory challenges of the prosecution. The burden was on the prosecutor to show neutral reasons for challenging all the black individuals so as not to be in violation of the Sixth and Fourteenth Amendments. The decision in *Batson v. Kentucky* (1986) is now settled law; the challenging party, usually the defendant in a criminal case, must be of a "cognizable racial group" and able to show that (usually) the prosecutor has used the allowed "peremptory challenges to remove . . . members of the defendant's race" (*Batson v. Kentucky*, 1986, Held: 3). Racial discrimination violates the Equal Protection Clause of the Fifth and Fourteenth Amendments to the U.S. Constitution. In 2016, the U.S. Supreme Court reaffirmed its decision in *Batson v. Kentucky* (1986) in stating that "The 'Constitution forbids striking even a single prospective juror for a discriminatory purpose'" (*Foster v. Chatman*, IIIA, para. 1).

Defendant Competency

For various purposes during the course of the proceedings, the defendant must be psychologically competent. We have already seen that if the defendant gave a confession, he or she had to have had the capacity to understand the *Miranda* warning and to know that certain constitutional rights were being waived prior to the confession being given and that this waiver was made voluntarily. Prior to trial, the defendant is given an opportunity to plead. As was seen, the issue of competency might come up if the plea is NGRI or even GBMI, which is a sort of hybrid between guilty and NGRI and very controversial (Kutys & Esterman, 2009). In the minority of jurisdictions that recognize GBMI and sustain the plea, the defendant could end up incarcerated, between a prison or jail sentence and a psychiatric commitment, for a greater length of time than a guilty plea would have mandated (Melville & Naimark, 2002). While that plea reverts back to competency at the time of the commission of the crime, other tests of competency are evaluated for the present time and purpose. Our justice system requires that the defendant be aware of and participatory in all facets of the proceedings. To that point, the Sixth Amendment states in part that the "accused" needs to be "informed of the nature and cause of the accusation." This is interpreted to mean that "informed" is synonymous with "understand."

To Stand Trial

Possibly the most common reason for hiring a forensic psychologist during the course of a criminal trial would be to evaluate the defendant's competency to stand trial (S. DeSales, personal communication, August 2012). A motion for a competency to stand trial hearing can come from either side or even the judge at any time during the course of the trial.[7] When the motion is made, it cannot be denied; the proceedings must stop, and a hearing must be scheduled (*Dusky v. United States*, 1960; see also 18 U.S.C 4244 for federal law). Although the standard has been refined by case law many times since (see, for example, *Indiana v. Edwards*, 2008), the landmark case that iterated a clear test for competency to stand trial was *Dusky v. United States* in 1960. In a brief unanimous opinion, the U.S. Supreme Court reversed the Eighth Circuit Court of Appeals (Ohio) that had affirmed Dusky's conviction and stated that the defendant is entitled to a full hearing when competency to stand trial is at issue, and that competency must be determined by the defendant's "ability to consult with his lawyer with a reasonable degree of rational understanding—and whether he has a rational as well as factual understanding of the proceedings against him" (18 U.S.C. 4241; *Dusky v. United States*, 1960, para. 2)

To Act as Own Attorney

Although the Sixth Amendment of the U.S. Constitution guarantees the right to an attorney for criminal defendants, some defendants want to act as their own attorneys (*Godinez v. Moran*, 1993). Case law is a bit more murky regarding whether the defendant should be able to waive his or her right to an attorney and what the standard should be if allowed. In 1993, the U.S. Supreme Court in *Godinez v. Moran* decided that if a criminal defendant was competent to stand trial, no higher standard was required for allowing the waiving of the constitutional right to an attorney. However, in 2008, in *Indiana v. Edwards*, the Supreme Court said a finding that the defendant is competent to stand trial was not enough to establish that the defendant was competent to waive the right to counsel. This makes sense, as the former is interpreted as the assertion of a constitutional right and the latter would be the rejecting of one.

Another issue that was more satisfactorily resolved in *Edwards* was the problem of commitment or institutionalization. Practically up until the decision in that case, defendants could be institutionalized indefinitely if found not competent to stand trial. The order was usually written so that the defendant was to be institutionalized until such time as he or she was competent to stand trial. Safeguards have now been put in place to make certain that these individuals cannot be institutionalized for longer than their sentence might have been if they had received a guilty verdict and that periodic evaluations must be conducted (*Indiana v. Edwards*, 2008; see also CA PC § 1370(c)(2)). Again, although psychologists do not and cannot give legal opinions, they must be so familiar with the legal process that their psychological evaluations are detailed enough to address the specific competencies at issue (APA, 2013; Rohlehr & Pinals, 2015).

Presentation of the Case and Defenses

Evidence

Although "evidence" is a term used in psychology and the law and has been used throughout the first three chapters (and will be more completely detailed in Chapter 5), a few more words about it are warranted as we proceed to the actual case presentation. As can be seen by the forensic report about Brendan Dassey's competence to waive his right against self-incrimination, what is presented during the course of a trial is the material, in whatever format, that will help the particular party. These presentations may be in the form

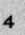

of testimony, documentation, or tangible items and are subject to admissibility by objection from the other party and court decision.

Order of Presentation

After an acceptable jury is empaneled, the prosecution presents first. The reasoning behind this is that the prosecution must prove the case beyond a reasonable doubt, and the defendant is innocent until proven guilty. The parties are first given an opportunity to make an opening statement. No evidence is required for this statement, and it is not required to make the statement. After opening statements, the prosecution presents its case through the various forms of evidence that are admissible, usually through testimony of witnesses. During this presentation, the defense is allowed to object to the evidence presented on various grounds, and the courts will rule as to whether the objection is sustained or overruled. After each witness is examined by the prosecution, the defense is allowed to cross-examine the witness. Recall from Chapter 3 that the case will be presented and judged in the best light for the defendant—therefore, the latitude allowed during cross-examination is much greater than that allowed during direct examination. Generally, whatever is raised during the direct examination can be challenged and expanded upon during the cross-examination. When all its testimony has been presented, the prosecution rests. In a criminal case, outside the hearing of the jury, the defense attorney will move to dismiss the case on the grounds that the prosecution did not prove its case beyond a reasonable doubt. Assuming the judge does not grant the dismissal, the next step is for the defense to present its case. Since the defendant is presumed innocent, the defense does not have to present a case and might rest; however, this would be most unusual. At this point, the burden of proof shifts to the defense as the presenting party, and the burden is to put reasonable doubt in the minds of the jurors (American Bar Association, 2017).

Expert Testimony

Although more will be said about expert testimony in Chapter 5, it is worth mentioning here in regard to the Jody Arias trial. There were few or no publicized issues regarding any unusual pretrial motions or jury selection, but during the course of her trial, at least two forensic mental health expert witnesses were called upon to help provide her with a defense. The results were quite controversial. The first mental health professional diagnosed Arias with post-traumatic stress disorder (PTSD), yet had not spent any face-to-face time with the defendant after she lied when she denied killing Travis Alexander (Lohr, 2013b). Upon cross-examination, the "expert" admitted to not writing down enough or correct information and not going back to the defendant to administer more tests or conduct a further interview after her DNA was found at the crime scene, and she confessed to having been there.

The second expert was a well-known domestic violence expert, who attempted to speak to the possibility that the defendant could have been abused, as she claimed in her own defense (Lohr, 2013a). While she spent a significant amount of time with Arias, Alyce LaViolette gave somewhat evasive testimony regarding the specifics of the alleged abuse perpetrated on Arias; what she ended up saying was that the defendant could have been a domestic violence victim (Weiner, Guerro, & Lustig, 2013). This testimony continued for 3 days, during which LaViolette mostly discussed the books and articles she had given to Arias about intimate partner violence (Weiner et al., 2013). The American Psychological Association's *Specialty Guidelines for Forensic Psychology* (2013) clearly state that competence and expertise go to knowledge regarding the case "at hand," not general knowledge about the subject matter (Introduction). LaViolette, however, is not a psychologist, forensic or otherwise. She has a master's degree in family therapy, and it is doubtful she belongs to the American Psychological Association (Harper, 2013).

Jury Instructions

Suggested jury instructions are provided to the judge by the attorneys from both sides. The judge, the trier of the law, then selects those provisions he or she deems most appropriate to the law at issue so the jury, as trier of the facts, can apply that law to the facts as they perceive them. Most appeals are based on what the appellant calls defective jury instructions or jury instructions in error. As was seen in *Elonis v. United*

States (2015) in Chapter 3, the Amicus Curiae brief expressed certainty the jury instructions given at Anthony Elonis's trial were erroneous and led to an incorrect verdict, and the U.S. Supreme Court agreed.

Although forensic psychologists do not have any direct input regarding jury instructions or any other law that is used, they do need to understand all facets of the trial (American Psychological Association, 2013; Gordon, 2006). For example, it is undisputed that George Zimmerman shot and killed Trayvon Martin in 2012. Trayvon Martin was a 17-year-old black teenager who was walking through the gate-guarded community where Zimmerman lived when Zimmerman, carrying a gun because of his neighborhood watch status, began following Martin. Zimmerman was not black and was told when he called 911 to return to his car and not follow the teenager. Zimmerman did not follow those instructions, and the exact ensuing events were vague. However, there was some evidence: Zimmerman had an open injury on the back of his head that required medical attention, and the victim was shot from close range in the stomach. During the trial, Zimmerman's attorney dragged a large piece of concrete into the courtroom and simulated a head being repeatedly banged on the concrete. The defense maintained that during the scuffle Martin was on top of Zimmerman banging his head on the concrete. Zimmerman stated Martin jumped him and reached for Zimmerman's gun, and Zimmerman shot him in self-defense. The trial created much controversy in 2013 when a six-woman jury acquitted Zimmerman.

I was teaching a course called *Law and Social Psychology* to two classes of doctoral students that summer, and the discussions were endless regarding Zimmerman's guilt. Because these students were preparing to be forensic psychologists, I spent a lot of time cautioning objectivity—not an easy task when so many were so certain there had been blatant prejudice on the part of the jurors. As soon as the verdict was announced, I knew I needed to meet my students with my own objectivity and present them with the jury instructions read in the case. The second legal lesson would be that due to the Fifth Amendment's statement about double jeopardy, the state of Florida could not appeal, and the defendant would not be punished for what most of these students considered murder. However, the instructions did provide an excellent example as a first lesson to show how the jury applied the facts to the law given to them by the judge (Jury Instructions for jurors in George Zimmerman murder trial, 2013).

Although Judge Nelson's instructions included the elements of second-degree murder and manslaughter, which were the crimes with which Zimmerman was charged, as well as other excuses for the commission of a homicide, the salient part of the instructions consisted of the instructions about self-defense, Zimmerman's defense. In Florida, "(a) person is justified in using deadly force if he reasonably believes that such force is necessary to prevent imminent death or great bodily harm to himself" (Jury instructions for jurors in George Zimmerman murder trial, 2013). Further, Judge Nelson instructed the jury that it was to consider only the circumstances at the time Zimmerman shot Martin. Of course, there were those who wanted to argue that the instructions were incorrect and those who flatly stated that Zimmerman was a liar. As to the former, the students were reminded that the jury instructions were repeated straight from Florida law regarding justifiable homicide, and the jury could only look to the facts as presented regarding the latter. They were reminded of Zimmerman's documented head injury and the defense strategy of bringing in the large piece of concrete. Martin was shot from the front at close range. While nobody agreed with the outcome, most of the students did understand how the jury came away with its verdict and learned the important lesson of objectivity required in the reporting of forensic psychologists.

Verdict and Judgment and Post-Trial Motions

Sometimes a jury cannot reach a unanimous verdict required in a criminal case. In that instance, the judge, usually after sending them back for further deliberation and/or individual questioning, can dismiss the jury and the case. If there is a verdict of not guilty, the trial court's job is also over, and the case is dismissed. If, however, the verdict is guilty, defense counsel has the opportunity to make a motion that asks the judge to enter judgment in opposition to the verdict. This would be extremely rarely granted, and the case would move on to judgment. When the judge enters the judgment, the jury's verdict becomes final.

Sentencing

Sentencing the guilty defendant becomes a separate proceeding from the actual trial phase, and a pre-sentencing investigation might ensue to help inform the court or a reconvened or newly convened jury on appropriate sentencing (American Bar Association, 2017). As closure for the Jody Arias saga, after her sentencing hearing ended twice in mistrials because jurors could not unanimously agree on the death penalty or life without the possibility of parole, she was finally sentenced to life without the possibility of parole in 2015 (Kiefer, 2015).

Death Penalty

Death penalty cases are of particular interest to psychologists. In states that allow capital punishment, the defense attorney will, of course, work to keep the client from getting that sentence. As will be seen by the illustrative cases, the law is settled that certain individuals cannot receive the death penalty. However, it will also become apparent that at least one of those cases might have caused more controversy than it resolved. As was noted earlier in this chapter, it is also settled law that even if the person has been correctly sentenced to death, the execution cannot be carried out if at the time of the execution the individual is not competent; he or she must understand the nature of and reason for the execution (Murray & Soroko, 1989).

Life Without the Possibility of Parole

Although the stated purpose of incarceration for criminals in the United States is both punishment and rehabilitation, some acts are deemed so heinous that the law provides the sentence of life without the possibility of parole (Benson, 2003). This is a particularly frequent sentence in states that do not have the death penalty.[8] However, as of 2012, juveniles are exempt from this sentence, regardless of the crime (*Miller v. Alabama*, 2012). In deciding that a sentence of life without the possibility of parole violated the Eighth Amendment's ban on cruel and unusual punishment, U.S. Supreme Court Justice Elena Kagan relied on an earlier case, *Roper v. Simmons* (2005) that is briefed below. Two cases of boys who were 14 years old when they committed their crimes were heard, with the only issue being whether their sentences violated the Eighth Amendment. The majority decided that based on the precedents—namely, that the Eighth Amendment prohibited juveniles from being sentenced to the death penalty (*Roper v. Simmons*, 2005) and from receiving a sentence of life without the possibility of parole if the crime did not involve a homicide (*Graham v. Florida*, 2010)—banning life without the possibility of parole even if a homicide is involved was the next logical step. Justice Kagan took language from the court's decision in *Roper* to state that punishment should be "graduated and proportioned" to be viewed according to "evolving standards of decency" (*Miller v. Alabama*, 2012, p. 6).

SPOTLIGHT ON CASES

Although many precedent-setting and some just plain interesting cases have been presented in this chapter, two more are worthy of review. Since *Roper v. Simmons* (2005) was mentioned as a precedent to *Miller v. Alabama* 7 years later, it appears here, followed by the earlier case of *Atkins v. Virginia* (2002)—the case on which Christopher Simmons based his appeal.

Roper v. Simmons (2005)

Facts: In 1993 at age 17, Christopher Simmons planned and perpetrated a murder. The fact that he was the instigator acting with intent was undisputed. With an accomplice, he had burglarized the house of Shirley Cook, who woke up and recognized him from an earlier incident. He decided to murder her by binding and gagging her and throwing her off a bridge to drown in the body of water below. Possibly because he had expressed certainty that he would get away with the murder due to his minority, he waived his right to an attorney and confessed when he was arrested.

Procedure: Simmons was tried as an adult in Missouri State Court and was convicted and sentenced to death. He then filed for postconviction relief in both state and federal courts. By the time those filings and decisions had run their course, the U.S. Supreme Court had decided *Atkins v. Virginia* (2002). Based on the Supreme Court's decision that mentally retarded individuals should not receive the death penalty (see the following case), Simmons argued that juveniles should not receive this punishment, either. The Missouri Supreme Court agreed and set aside the death sentence, giving Simmons life without the possibility of parole. Donald Roper, the named petitioner and superintendent of the correctional center, appealed the state court's decision based on the belief that the Eighth Amendment does not prohibit the execution of minors.

Issue: Does the death penalty violate the Eighth and Fourteenth Amendments when applied to juveniles?

Rule: The majority quoted many psychology studies as well as earlier editions of the *Diagnostic and Statistical Manual of Mental Disorders* (*DSM*; American Psychiatric Association, 2013) and looked to the general trend in state punishment to decide that executing minors is cruel and unusual punishment and violative of the Due Process Clause of the Fourteenth Amendment.

Holding: The judgment of the Missouri Supreme Court was affirmed. The Eighth and Fourteenth Amendments "forbid" a death penalty sentence for a perpetrator who was under 18 at the time of the crime.

Judgment: Reversed for Roper.

Atkins v. Virginia (2002)

Unfortunately, *Atkins v. Virginia*, which was the case that set precedent for *Roper v. Simmons* (2005) and *Miller v. Alabama* (2012), did not clarify specifically who could and could not be executed when cognitive competence is the issue.

Facts: Daryl Atkins and an accomplice robbed and murdered Nesbitt. They were armed with semiautomatic weapons and shot their victim eight times. Although some parts of the crime were on video, the actual shooter was unknown. Because Atkin's accomplice proved to be the more articulate of the two, his version of the crime, which claimed that Atkins was the shooter, was believed. Prior to the sentencing phase of the case, Atkins underwent an evaluation by a forensic psychologist, who reported that he was mentally retarded (this is the court's term) after interviewing him, collecting background information, and administering standardized tests.

Procedure: Atkins was tried and convicted in Virginia under state law. His first sentencing hearing turned out to be procedurally faulty, and during the second resentencing hearing, the state presented an expert rebuttal witness to the original evaluator who stated Daryl had antisocial personality disorder and was of at least average intelligence (*Atkins v. Virginia*, 2002).[9] Atkins was again sentenced to death. Because two justices strongly dissented in the majority opinion in the state court, the U.S. Supreme Court agreed to review the case.

Issue: Does the execution of mentally retarded individuals violate the Eighth Amendment in interpreting its prohibition under an "evolving standard of decency?"(*Atkins v. Virginia*, 2002, part IV, para. 7)?

Rule: Aside from the national consensus about executing the mentally retarded that is evolving, and Eighth Amendment prohibitions, there is no reason to assume that executing mentally retarded individuals will serve any legal or societal purpose.

Holding: Mentally retarded individuals will no longer be sentenced to execution; however, it is up to the states to define mental retardation based on Eighth Amendment requirements.

Judgment: Reversed for Atkins

Epilogue: Although most jurisdictions seem to recognize that mental retardation needs to be defined by more than an IQ score with an arbitrary cutoff point, the state of Florida had a statute that did just that, stating that only an IQ score of under 70 would be considered mental retardation. The state's argument was that the *Atkins* decision allowed the states to define mental retardation any way they decided was appropriate. In 2014, in *Hall v. Florida*, the U.S. Supreme Court ruled that while a state could set an IQ score anywhere it wanted to judge mental retardation, it was unconstitutional to do so without other criteria such as looking to the individual's adaptive functioning. In coming to its decision, the court frequently referenced an Amicus Curiae brief filed by the American Psychological Association in 2013 in support of Freddie Lee Hall.

FOCUS ON CAREERS

ADAM YERKE

Dr. Adam Yerke has been a licensed psychologist since 2008, having received his doctor of psychology (PsyD) degree from the California School of Professional Psychology. Of more relevance, he is certified by the state of California to not only evaluate and treat sex offenders, but also train clinicians and students to do the same. California's certification process is rigorous and demanding; few, if any, would disagree that the evaluation process requires that only those who understand and comply with the laws and regulations should be in a position to determine the risks involved in declaring a sex offender fit for release, parole, or probation.

Many literally recoil at the mention of the phrase "sexually violent predator" or even the more benign "sexual offender." What Dr. Yerke knows and teaches is that sex offenders, although referred to as a group, cannot realistically or practically be grouped together. Their offenses cover a broad range from public exposure, to viewing child pornography, to rape of adults or children. Within even those general categories, the law and psychology define more specific parafilias and parafilic disorders (American Psychiatric Association, 2013), misdemeanors (minor crimes punishable by fine or jail time, or both), and/or felonies (punishable by fine or prison time, or both). Although a minority of sex offenders can be classified as having parafilias (i.e., unusual sexual desires), Dr. Yerke recognizes an increased interest in what motivates and drives their behaviors. At times, Dr. Yerke's role is to visit a state hospital where sexual offenders have been civilly committed to evaluate them for fitness for release or to treat them. He does this through his work at a forensic agency that contracts with the state to evaluate and treat sex offenders who have been convicted and are required to get treatment.

(continued)

(continued)

Adam Yerke has always worked in what might be called (not by him) the darker side of society. Throughout his graduate school education, he worked at outpatient facilities treating clients with substance abuse issues. For his predoctoral internship, he was offered an opportunity to work with sex offenders and was gratified to be able to take advantage of the experience. He quickly learned that the general public and even some graduate students have much misinformation about sex offenders, including their behaviors, assessment, and treatment. However, he also soon realized that his state, California, was doing things correctly through the creation of evidence-based programs within which he wanted to practice. Dr. Yerke would certainly be considered an expert in training and supervising others to evaluate and treat sex offenders, but he is also an expert in sex offender management and evaluation, a published author, a professor, and a lecturer. He has expertise in treating addictions, anxiety, and other psychological disorders, and is a certified independent practitioner with the California State Sex Offender Management Board as well as chair of the California Coalition on Sex Offending (COSO).

TRISHA ELLOYAN

From Nevada to New York, back to Nevada, and finally to California, **Dr. Trisha Elloyan** has pursued her interest in the practice of forensic psychology both educationally and experientially. Realizing she would not reach her professional goals with a bachelor's degree in psychology and indulging in her lifelong love of the law, Dr. Elloyan went to New York and received a master's degree in forensic psychology from a highly regarded criminal justice program. Upon returning to her native Nevada, she went to work in the courts, administering a specialty court program for 6 years. Unfortunately, she was not professionally satisfied with her role in the system. As far as she was concerned, she was an

(continued)

(*continued*)

"onlooker" and not involved with the individuals for whom the court was established. Dr. Elloyan knew that to achieve her goal of program development for offenders. she would need her doctorate. Her motivation was a desire to "understand and treat" the psychological reasons behind criminal behavior. To her, this was the way she could serve to help "break the cycle" of the unlawful behavior in which so many engaged. In her own words, she wanted to learn how to be "proactive" rather than "reactive."

During her doctoral education, Dr. Elloyan worked with paroled and on-probation sex offenders in an outpatient treatment facility, and with juvenile offenders on probation. She completed her predoctoral clinical training at a state prison. She continues there as an employee finishing her postdoctoral hours with plans to continue her career as a forensic psychologist at the prison. While the population with whom she works at the prison are inmates, they all have mental health diagnoses and are technically referred to as Level 2, enhanced outpatients. These inmates are given the highest level of mental healthcare except for those in need of crisis intervention. They require 10 hours of services each week, and Dr. Elloyan currently services 24 individuals who attend two group sessions each week for aggression replacement therapy.

Although Dr. Elloyan believes that services for the mentally ill are improving, at least at her facility, she sees much room for improvement and hopes to eventually be in a position there to create and develop programs and services for the needy population. She would also like to expand her work to include creating and developing alternative sentencing programs in the courts, especially programming for specific types of mentally ill inmates and/or paroled mentally ill inmates.

To illustrate her point, and to further understand the work that forensic psychologists such as Dr. Yerke and she do, Dr. Elloyan relates the following story: An inmate whom she treats. who is obviously developmentally delayed, was originally arrested for public exposure. He had urinated on a public

(*continued*)

(continued)

street. His crime was a misdemeanor, but because it is considered a sex offense, the court ordered him to register as a sexual offender in California. For whatever reason (Dr. Elloyan believes he did not understand the requirement), he neglected to register. He was then arrested for failure to register as a sex offender, a felony, and sentenced to 3 years in prison.

For this man and so many others like him, Drs. Yerke and Elloyan are there to evaluate, treat, and try to create change. Their specialized training and dedication to their work make a difference not only for these individuals, but for all those with whom they come in contact, our justice system, and our communities.

IN THE NEWS

The topics covered in this chapter give rise to many potentially newsworthy stories. If the sheer number of stories is any indication of potential work opportunities for forensic psychologists, it is highly doubtful there will be enough of them to cover the need. In March 2017, the U.S. Supreme Court set aside a death penalty sentence for a convicted murderer who had been on death row in Texas since 1980 (Savage, 2017). The majority agreed that Texas had used outdated standards to sentence him to death. In a span of less than 10 days, two more relevant stories were in the news: A former basketball coach pleaded not guilty to sexually abusing a 14-year-old girl, a felony (Kohli, 2017), and an accused murderer decided to plead NGRI to the murder of a doctor (Puente, 2017). Both crimes occurred in Southern California, and there are certainly issues in both that will require the services of forensic psychologists.

These three news stories are not unusual in the United States, and many more could be mentioned. However, a case that has been in the news and is most unusual bears a deeper reading. Michelle Carter was 17 years old when she and her friend Conrad Roy III finally finished exchanging thousands of text messages in 2014. The text messages were interpreted as the communication between two troubled teenagers that began in 2012, when Michelle was encouraging Conrad to seek treatment (Seelye & Bidgood, 2017). By 2014, however, Michelle was encouraging Conrad, who had attempted suicide previously, to actually do it. On the day he died, according to Michelle's own statement to a friend, they had stopped texting and were talking on the phone. When Conrad told Michelle he had filled his truck with lethal carbon monoxide but had exited the truck, Michelle told him to get back in and finally commit suicide.

Her trial was in front of a judge only, as she had waived her right to a jury trial after being charged with involuntary manslaughter under state law. In Massachusetts, involuntary manslaughter is an unlawful killing unintentionally caused by the defendant's wanton or reckless conduct (Tarantola, 2017). Although there is much controversy surrounding not only Carter's arrest, but also her role in the suicide, in reading his decision, the judge made it clear that Carter's behavior during that last phone call provided his reasoning for finding her guilty. Her behavior in telling Roy to reenter the car and in not helping him was reckless and resulted in her unintentional killing of him (Seelye & Bidgood, 2017). On August 3, 2017, Michelle Carter was sentenced to 2.6 years in prison and 5 years probation (Boroff, 2017).

This case brings to mind the earlier suicide of Tyler Clementi. In 2011, his Rutgers roommate, Dharun Ravi, and a friend video recorded Clementi having sex in their room with another man and video streamed it. As a result, Clementi killed himself. Ravi was charged with several counts of intimidation and criminal invasion of privacy under New Jersey law and was convicted of some of them. In 2012, Ravi was sentenced to 30 days in jail and 3 years probation. He appealed, and in 2016, his conviction was overturned for several reasons, including the repeal of several laws under which he had been convicted (*State of New Jersey v. Dharun Ravi*, 2016). Although as with Michelle Carter, the development of social media probably led to what both courts called "cyberbullying," the opinion in Ravi's appeal made it very clear that Ravi was not charged with or considered legally responsible for Clementi's death (*State of New Jersey v. Dharun Ravi*, 2016). Michelle Carter's case is a first in this area, but with social media becoming an everyday way of life, teenage suicide on the rise, and the term "cyberbullying" signaling a new form of harassment, there are bound to be many more (*State of New Jersey v. Dharun Ravi*, 2016; Tarantola, 2017).

SUMMARY

The title of this chapter laid the foundation for the topics that would be covered regarding forensic psychologists' involvement in criminal matters. The range of topics is so broad that the best approach was to trace the criminal case from its inception—that is, the discovery of a crime—through sentencing. Along the way, those components of the case that would most likely involve the services of forensic psychologists were highlighted. Because many of the criminally related topics in forensic psychology are collateral to the actual trial progression, and because forensic psychologists may be called in for criminally related matters that are not necessarily criminal, those issues were also addressed at appropriate junctures.

While all types of crimes and punishment were covered through case law, news reports, journal articles, and interviews, a new crime was also discussed. In the decades to come, understanding and deciding cases related to "suicide by remote technology" will undoubtedly create work, research, and joint projects for forensic psychologists engaged in practice and research, attorneys, and the courts.

DISCUSSION QUESTIONS

1. The NGRI plea basically tells the court the defendant committed the act, but should not be held liable because he or she could not form the requisite intent. How do you think California (and other jurisdictions) might reconcile allowing the dual pleas of not guilty (didn't do it) and NGRI by the same defendant for the same act?

2. Dr. Yerke says the majority of sex offenders do not have a *DSM* diagnosis. Do you think the behavior of the majority, then, has a common point of motivation? Are all sex offenders the same in regard to their offending behavior? Should they all be punished in the same way?

3. Dr. Elloyan says one of her goals in her chosen profession would be to be more involved in program planning for inmates. Discuss what kinds of programs might be helpful or appropriate for prison inmates.

4. *Roper v. Simmons* (2005) was very clear that a person under the age of 18 at the time of committing a crime cannot be sentenced to death. That means if two perpetrators commit exactly the same crime and one is 17 years and 11 months at the time and the other is 18 the day before, the latter could receive the death penalty. As a forensic psychologist called in by defense counsel, how could you make an argument for the 18-year-old's life?

NOTES

1. The definition of homicide is commonly misunderstood among nonlaw enforcement and other nonlegal professionals. Homicide is not always a criminal matter (see, for example, Li, Joutsijoki, Laurikkala, Siermala, & Juhola, 2015). It is undisputed that a homicide has occurred if an individual causes the accidental death of another person, or if law enforcement legally kills a perpetrator. These are still killings of a human being by another human being.

2. For example, there may be a plea bargain if the evidence is so strong and obvious that the defendant knows there almost has to be a guilty verdict, or as a way to remove the death penalty as a possibility if there is a guilty verdict.

3. As of August 23, 2017, Scott DeKraai was sentenced to eight consecutive life sentences without the possibility of parole.

4. See, for example, Bartol and Bartol (2015) and/or Syllabus/Course Map/ catalogue description: The Chicago School of Professional Psychology Introduction to Forensic Psychology (2009–2017) FO 610, PF 610, www .thechicagoschool.edu.

5. Generally, the *Miranda* warning consists of four statements:

   1. You have the right to remain silent.
   2. Anything you say can and will be used against you in a court of law.
   3. You have the right to an attorney.
   4. If you cannot afford an attorney, one will be appointed for you (*Miranda* rights and the Fifth Amendment, n.d.).

6. The other would be "not guilty."
7. This is one of the few times a judge is allowed his or her own motion during the course of the trial. The correct name for the judge's motion is a "sua sponte" motion.
8. As of 2014, 18 states did not have the death penalty (see https://www .washingtonpost.com/news/post-nation/wp/2014/04/30/there-are-18-states-without-the-death-penalty-a-third-of-them-have-banned-it-since-2007/?utm_term=.7715bea14021).
9. The first evaluator found Atkins' IQ to be 59, which is at least two standard deviations below average. The case does not reflect the credentials or the actual evaluation of the second evaluator.

REFERENCES

18 U.S.C. 4241 (1948).

18 U.S.C. 4244 (1949).

Allen, F. A. (1962). The rule of the American Law Institute's Model Penal Code. *Marquette Law Review, 45*(4), 494–505.

American Bar Association. (2017). *How courts work.* Retrieved from https:// www.americanbar.org/groups/public_education/resources/law_ related_education_network/how_courts_work/juryselect.html

American Psychiatric Association. (2013). *Diagnostic and statistical manual of mental disorders* (5th ed.). Washington, DC: Author.

American Psychological Association. (2013). Specialty guidelines for forensic psychology. *American Psychologist, 68*(1), 7–19. doi:10.1037/a0029889

Atkins v. Virginia, 536 U.S. 304 (2002).

Attanasio, P., & McGraw, P. (Creators & Writers). (2016). *Bull* [Television series]. United States: Amblin Television.

Bartol, C. R., & Bartol, A. M. (2015). *Introduction to forensic psychology: Research and application* (5th ed.). Los Angeles, CA: Sage.

Batson v. Kentucky, 476 U.S. 79 (1986).

Benson, E. (2003). Rehabilitate or punish? *Monitor on Psychology, 43*(7), 46.

Berman, S. J. (2017a). The basics of a plea bargain. *Nolo.* Retrieved from http://www.nolo.com/legal-encyclopedia/the-basics-plea-bargain.html

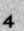

Berman, S. J. (2017b). Homicide: Murder and manslaughter. *Nolo*. Retrieved from http://www.nolo.com/legal-encyclopedia/homicide-murder-manslaughter-32637.html

Blackwood, H. L., Rogers, R., Steadham, J. A., & Fiduccia, C. E. (2015). Investigating *Miranda* waiver decisions: An examination of the rational consequences. *International Journal of Law and Psychiatry, 42–43,* 11–18.

Boroff, D. (2017, August 3). Michelle Carter sentenced to 2-1/2 years for sending boyfriend texts encouraging suicide. *New York Daily News*. Retrieved from http://www.nydailynews.com/news/crime/michelle-carter-sentenced-2-1-2-years-suicide-texts-article-1.3381578

Bousfield, R. M., & Merrett, R. (1843). *Report of the trial of Daniel M'naughton at the Central Criminal court.* London, UK: Henry Renshaw.

Burden of Proof. (2017). Current application of the insanity defense. *FindLaw*. Retrieved from http://criminal.findlaw.com/criminal-procedure/current-application-of-the-insanity-defense.html

California Evidence Code § 522 (2015).

Chen, S. (2009). What does "person of interest" mean? Nothing. *CNN*. Retrieved from http://www.cnn.com/2009/CRIME/09/17/yale.person.of.interest/index.html#cnnSTCText

Coffin v. United States, 1856 U.S. 432 (1895).

Crimes & Punishments, CA Penal Code §§ 25-29.8 (2016).

Demos, M., & Ricciara, L. (Producers). (2015). *Making a murderer* [Television series]. Manitowoc, WI: Netflix.

Dusky v. United States, 362 U.S. 402 (1960).

Elonis v. United States, 135 S. Ct. 2001 (2015).

Flores, A. (2014, May 2). Seal Beach mass shooting suspect Scott Dekraai now a convicted killer. *Los Angeles Times*. Retrieved from http://www.latimes.com/local/la-me-0503-seal-beach-killer-20140503-story.html

Foster v. Chatman, 136 S. Ct. 1737 (2016).

Frumkin, I. B., Lally, S. J., & Sexton, J. E. (2012). The Grisso tests for assessing understanding and appreciation of *Miranda* warnings with a forensic sample. *Behavioral Sciences and the Law, 30*(6), 673–692.

Fry, H. (2017, August 22). Jury begins deliberating sanity of man convicted of killing Newport Beach urologist. *Daily Pilot*. Retrieved from http://www.latimes.com/socal/daily-pilot/news/tn-dpt-me-elkus-verdict-update-20170822-story.html

Godinez v. Moran, 509 U.S. 389 (1993).

Goldstein, N. E. S., Zelle, H., & Grisso, T. (2012). *Miranda rights comprehension instruments (MRCI): Manual for juvenile and adult evaluations.* Sarasota, FL: Professional Resource Press.

Gomez, M. M. (2016). *Jury trials outside in.* Boulder, CO: National Institute for Trial Advocacy.

Gordon, R. H. (2006). *Exhibit 231: Brendan Dassey psych evaluation.* Retrieved from http://www.stevenaverycase.org/wp-content/uploads/2016/01/Trial-Exhibit-231-Brendan-Dassey-Psych-Evaluation-11-10-2006.pdf

Graham v. Florida, 560 U.S. 48 (2010).

Grisso, T. (1980). Juveniles' capacities to waive *Miranda* rights: An empirical analysis. *California Law Review, 68*(6), 1134–1166.

Hall v. Florida, Brief for defendant Freddie Lee Hall as Amicus Curiae, *Hall v. Florida* 134 S.Ct.1986 (2014).

Harper, J. (2013, April 11). The mobbing of Alyce LaViolette. *Psychology Today.* Retrieved from https://www.psychologytoday.com/blog/beyond-bullying/201304/the-mobbing-alyce-laviolette

Homicide definition. (2013). *Findlaw.* Retrieved from http://files.findlaw.com/pdf/criminal/criminal.findlaw.com_criminal-charges_homicide-definition.pdf

Indiana v. Edwards, 544 U.S. 164 (2008).

Jury Instructions for jurors in George Zimmerman murder trial. (2013, July 12). [Video]. Retrieved from https://www.youtube.com/watch?v=lvkaMA9q6CE

Kiefer, M. (2015, April 13). Jodi Arias sentenced to natural life in prison. *USA Today.* Retrieved from https://www.usatoday.com/story/news/nation/2015/04/13/jodi-arias-sentencing/25691575/

Kohli, S. (2017, July 3). Former Hacienda Heights basketball coach pleads not guilty to sexually abusing a 14-year-old student. *Los Angeles Times.* Retrieved from http://www.latimes.com/local/education/la-essential-education-updates-southern-former-hacienda-heights-basketball-1499091046-htmlstory.html

Kutys, J., & Esterman, J. (2009). Guilty but mentally ill (GBMI) vs. not guilty by reason of insanity (NGRI). *Jury Expert, 21*(6), 28–31. Retrieved from http://thejuryexpert.com/wp-content/uploads/TJEVol21Num6_Nov2009.pdf

Lehmann, J. K., & Smith, J. B. (2013). A multidimensional examination of jury composition, trial outcomes, and attorney preferences. *Working Paper.* Retrieved from http://www.uh.edu/~jlehman2/papers/lehmann_smith_jurycomposition.pdf

Li, X., Joutsijoki, H., Laurikkala, J., Siermala, M., & Juhola, M. (2015). Homicide and its social context: Analysis using the self-organizing map. *Applied Artificial Intelligence, 29,* 382–401. doi:10.1080/08839514.2015.1016774

Lilienfeld, S. O., & Arkowitz, H. (2011, January). The insanity verdict on trial. *Scientific American.* Retrieved from https://www.scientificamerican.com/article/the-insanity-verdict-on-trial

Lohr, D. (2013a, April 2). Jodi Arias domestic violence expert Alyce LaViolette to resume testimony. *Huffpost*. Retrieved from http://www.huffingtonpost .com/2013/04/02/jodi-arias-trial-live-blog-day-39_n_2999563.html

Lohr, D. (2013b, March 18). Richard Samuels, key witness in Jodi Arias trial admits to "oversight." *Huffpost*. Retrieved from http://www.huffingtonpost .com/2013/03/18/jodi-arias-defense-expert-cross-examination-richard-samuels_n_2904063.html

Louszko, A., Torres, I., Effron, L., & Newman, B. (2016). *Making a Murderer*: The complicated argument over Brendan Dassey's confession. *ABC News*. Retrieved from http://nymag.com/scienceofus/2016/01/science-behind-brendan-dasseys-confession.html

McLaughlin, E. C. (2013, May 8). Haven't been following the Jody Arias trial? Read this. *CNN*. Retrieved from http://www.cnn.com/2013/05/04/us/jodi-arias-primer/index.html

Melville, J. D. (2002). Punishing the insane: The verdict of guilty but mentally ill. *Journal of the Academy of Psychiatry and the Law, 30,* 553–555.

Miller v. Alabama, 567 U.S. 460 (2012).

"*Miranda* rights" and the Fifth Amendment. (n.d.). *FindLaw*. Retrieved from http://criminal.findlaw.com/criminal-rights/miranda-rights-and-the-fifth-amendment.html

Miranda v. Arizona, 384 U.S. 436 (1966).

Murray, F., & Soroko, L., (Producers) & Pearce, R. (Director). (1989). *Dead man out* [Motion picture]. Canada: IM Global & WWE Studios.

People v. Wheeler, 22 Cal. 3d 258 (1978).

Pleadings & Proceedings before Trial. CA Penal Code § 1026 (2016).

Puente, K. (2017, July 27). Trial begins for man accused of killing Newport Beach doctor over medical procedure. *Los Angeles Times*, p. A1.

Rangel, D. (2015, October). *Ethics for criminal law attorneys*. Presentation at the State Bar of California 88th Annual Meeting Anaheim, California.

Replogle, J. (2017, July 4). Orange County Sheriff to testify in jailhouse snitch scandal. *Crime & Justice KPCC* [Radio broadcast]. Retrieved from http://www.scpr.org/news/2017/07/04/73504/orange-county-sheriff-to-testify-in-jailhouse-snit/

Rogers, R., Rogstad, J. E., Gillard, N. D., Blackwood, H. L., Drogin, E. Y., & Shuman, D. W. (2010). "Everyone knows their *Miranda* rights": Implicit assumption and countervailing evidence. *Psychology, Public Policy, & Law, 16,* 300–317.

Rohlehr, L. N., & Pinals, D. A. (2015). Competency to waive right to counsel. *Journal of the American Academy of Psychiatry and the Law Online, 43*(3), 385–387.

Roper v. Simmons, 543 U.S. 551 (2005).

State of New Jersey v. Dharun Ravi, No. A-4667-11T1 (2016).

Savage, D. G. (2017, March 29). Supreme Court lifts killer's death sentence. *Los Angeles Times*, p. A7.

Seelye, K. Q., & Bidgood, J. (2017, June 16). Guilty verdict for young woman who urged friend to kill himself. *New York Times*. Retrieved from https://www.nytimes.com/2017/06/16/us/suicide-texting-trial-michelle-carter-conrad-roy.html

Shaw, J. (2016, January 18). Making a memory of murder. *Scientific American*. Retrieved from https://blogs.scientificamerican.com/mind-guest-blog/making-a-memory-of-murder/

Singal, J. (2016, January 11). The science behind Brendan Dassey's agonizing confession in *Making a Murderer*. *Science of Us*. Retrieved from http://nymag.com/scienceofus/2016/01/science-behind-brendan-dasseys-confession.html

Tarantola, A. (2017, June 22). Death by text: How the Michelle Carter case will impact free speech. *Engadget*. Retrieved from https://www.engadget.com/2017/06/22/you-may-be-jailed-for-telling-someone-to-die-in-a-fire

Tedder-King, A., & Marinakis, C. (2016). Cut the bull: What can trial consultants really do? *Litigation Insights*. Retrieved from http://litigationinsights.com/jury-consulting/bull-cbs-trial-consultants-really-do/

Thompson, A., & Dirr, A. (2017, June 23). Conviction of "Making a Murderer" defendant, Brendan Dassey overturned. *USA Today*. Retrieved from https://www.usatoday.com/story/life/tv/2017/06/23/conviction-making-murderer-defendant-brendan-dassey-overturned/103132758/

Weiner, A. H., Guerra, E., & Lustig, M. (Producers). (2013). *Jodi Arias expert witness gets grilled in & out of court with Loni Coombs*. [Video]. Available from https://www.google.com/search?q=alyce+laviolette+biography&oq=alyce+laviolette+cv&aqs=chrome.1.69i57j0l2.17905j0j8&sourceid=chrome&ie=UTF-8

Williams v. Florida, 399 U.S. 78 (1970).

The Forensic Psychologist's Role in Civil Cases: Experts, Juries, and Research

OVERVIEW

After several years of interviewing potential forensic psychology students and answering questions at professional workshops and presentations, it sometimes seems to me as if most of the interest in forensic psychology is directed to the forensic psychologist's role in criminal proceedings (hence the length of the previous chapter!). However, the role of the forensic psychologist in civil matters is varied and far-reaching. This chapter describes various roles of the forensic psychologist as he or she provides **expert testimony** in civil cases, consults for civil **jury trials**, and assesses individuals for **competency**.[1] The focus of the cases might be **breach of contract** or various types of **torts**, including **product liability, professional malpractice,** and other forms of **negligence,** as well as **intentional torts;** these cases are included here not so much because of their subject matter, but because of their relevance to the process of the legal system and the work of the forensic psychologist. Since the U.S. legal system is a common law system, much of how psychology and the law work together is best illustrated by case law (see Chapter 4). Aside from the specific reason for employment in certain cases, the forensic psychologist is trained to discover **malingering,** a term used in psychology to describe deceptive behavior by the malingerer for his or her personal/legal gain (American Psychiatric Association, 2013).

Therefore, not only will the background and legal foundation for expert testimony be explained through case law in this chapter, but cases will also illustrate the various legal terms, how they work, and how the work of the forensic psychologist helps in establishing credible **evidence** in civil matters. As discussed in Chapter 2, courts operate within certain legal boundaries; they may set their own standards but are bound by the laws of the jurisdictions in which they sit. Two cases decided exactly 70 years apart provide the law for allowing expert testimony to be admitted when relevant. Every forensic psychology student needs to be familiar with *Frye v. United States* (1923) and *Daubert v. Merrell Dow Pharmaceuticals* (1993). *Romano v. Steelcase* (2010) is a product liability case that illustrates the impact of social media and the possibility of exposing malingering. Although a half-century old, *Dillon v. Legg* (1968) remains relevant as a civil case that not only illustrates the merger of psychology and the law, but more specifically established negligent infliction of emotional distress as a civil cause of action. It must also be remembered that when competency is challenged in a criminal case (see Chapter 4), its existence for a particular purpose will be determined in a civil proceeding.

Finally, the specific role of an expert witness is discussed through a profile of Dr. Jay Finkelman, along with a civil case whose outcome may have turned because of Dr. Finkelman's testimony. In fact, the profile and case example could well provide yet another area of civil law for the potential forensic psychologist to contemplate.

HOW IT WORKS

Background

While criminal law is about guilt and potential deprivation of freedom or even life, civil litigation is about liability and money. This difference is what explains why the burden of proof is reduced from beyond a reasonable doubt to usually a preponderance of the evidence, or to the somewhat higher standard of clear and convincing evidence. The best way to explain this difference is to go back over 20 years to two cases involving the same set of circumstances.

In 1994, Nicole Brown Simpson and Ron Goldman were stabbed to death in front of her home. Her former husband, O. J. Simpson, was arrested and tried for the murders. During the course of the trial, the prosecution presented **testimonial** and **physical** evidence to prove its case beyond a reasonable doubt, and the defendant's attorneys did their job of attempting to put reasonable doubt into the juror's minds throughout the case (Ito, 1995). Judge Ito's (1995) jury instructions defined reasonable doubt for the jurors and explained they had to look at the evidence in the best light for the defendant. Reasonable doubt, he explained, "is that state of the case which, after the entire comparison and consideration of all the evidence, leaves the minds of the jurors in that condition that they cannot say they feel an abiding conviction of the truth of the charge" (para. 29). The 12-member jury did not find the defendant guilty beyond a reasonable doubt.

After the acquittal of O. J. Simpson, the families filed wrongful death and other civil actions against him. In these cases, the plaintiffs' burden of proof was to show by a preponderance of the evidence that the defendant was responsible for the deaths of the victims (Simon, 1997). Although in a civil proceeding in California, only nine of the 12 jurors need agree, the jury returned a unanimous verdict of liability against the defendant and later awarded the plaintiffs millions of dollars in damages (Ayres, 1997). Although both verdicts were controversial at the time, and are still debated by some, the circumstances that led to the two trials provide a clear picture of how burdens of proof actually work in the courtroom.

Presentation/Admissibility of Evidence

While the forensic psychologist may participate at every phase of civil litigation, certain aspects are more commonly understood and utilized among the legal professionals and lay public (Gomez, 2013). All litigation relies on the evidence presented, including both the admissibility of that evidence and the weight given to it. Generally, all **relevant evidence** is admissible unless its **prejudicial effect** outweighs its **probative value** (Federal Rules of Evidence 401–403). Further, evidence may be testimonial, physical, and **documentary**, as well as **direct** or **circumstantial evidence**. Unless challenged by the other side, all evidence is admissible' when evidence is challenged, the judge decides as to its admissibility (Schweitzer & Saks, 2009).

In a breach of contract case, for example, the written contract would be direct, documentary evidence. For the sake of illustration, assume the contract was between a buyer and seller for the purchase of 5,000 pencils at a dollar apiece. When the pencils were delivered, the buyer refused to pay based on the appearance of the pencils—they were only 4 inches long. The seller sued the buyer because the pencils were custom made for the buyer with the buyer's company logo. The buyer defended on the grounds that he expected pencils of at least 7 inches in length, as was the custom of the trade. The direct documentary evidence (the contract) did not specify the length of the pencils. The seller offered the circumstantial physical evidence of 4-inch pencils that had been made for a dozen other companies. The buyer, in turn, offered the expert testimony, also circumstantial, of a pencil manufacturer whose credentials were unchallenged as the largest pencil manufacturer in the country. She stated her company had never manufactured a pencil shorter than 7 inches, and this was the usual length of a pencil (Uniform Commercial Code, 2001). The seller offered the testimony of a witness who was present at the signing and swore the seller gave the buyer every opportunity to ask any questions and alter any terms of the contract prior to signing. Assuming all of the proffered evidence is admissible and the parties proceed to trial, the next step would be jury selection.

Weight of the Evidence

Once selected, it would be the jurors' job as the triers of fact to determine how much weight, or credibility, each of these pieces of evidence should be given in making their final determination. Of course, in 2018 a $5,000 case is unlikely to reach a trial stage and certainly would not require the expertise of a forensic psychologist, but the example serves to illustrate how the services of the forensic psychologist might be utilized.

First, while the expert whose testimony is offered is a manufacturer and not a psychologist, the psychologist who understands what the court and/or jury is listening and looking for when an expert is testifying might well brief the witness and the attorney about questions to ask, effective dress, and nonverbal behavior. In addition, the forensic psychologist will be well versed in the order in which questions need to be asked and answered. Juries are known to be susceptible to what are called the primacy and recency effects, retaining the first information related versus retaining the last information related, respectively (Aronson, 2012).

Next, the eyewitness will require some counseling. The forensic psychologist has read the literature, and possibly contributed to it, and knows what jurors need to hear. While eyewitness testimony has a controversial history regarding its (lack of) accuracy, research shows that the more confidence the witness displays, the more credibility the jury perceives (Leippe, Eisenstadt, Rauch & Seib, 2004).[2] A recent meta-analysis by John Wixted and Gary Wells (2017) concluded that at least in criminal matters, if the identification process presented by law enforcement was "fair" and objective, there was a strong correlation between the confidence of the eyewitness and the accuracy of the identification (p. 20).

Special Purposes in General

The purpose or purposes for which an expert might be consulted are varied and often not predictable. Although much of what follows is as applicable to a criminal proceeding as a civil proceeding, it focuses on some of the more common reasons a forensic psychologist might be called upon during the course of a civil proceeding. The cases that follow the explanations are highligted because they are either precedent setting, illustrative of the construct, or both.

Witness Credibility

Just as psychologists are guided by ethical standards, attorneys have codes of professional responsibility that delineate the standards by which they practice (American Bar Association, 2002; American Psychological Association, 2013, 2017). Whether the code of ethical conduct is provided by the state or the American Bar Association, the provisions are similar: Counsel cannot coach a witness to the extent that there is the appearance of deception or withholding the truth (see, for example, American Bar Associationt, 2002; *California Rules of Professional Conduct*, 2017; Grodsky, 2012). However, attorneys agree witnesses need preparation for their testimony to be credible to a jury (Grodsky, 2012). An interesting study was conducted by an attorney and two trial consultants, both with doctorate degrees, after they interviewed a panel of jurors in an attempt to discover the impact the attorney's discrediting of a witness had on the jury's verdict (Stuhan, Gomez, & Wolfe, 2007). The attorney had shown that the witness testified differently on the stand than he had in an earlier deposition, and was proud that he had impeached the witness's credibility with a **prior inconsistent statement** that he was certain had a strong impact on the jury's decision. What he found was that the jurors believed the witness made an honest mistake, and the inconsistency was not of major importance in their minds (Stuhan et al., 2007).

Stuhan et al. (2007) then collected data from 810 mock jurors representing at least 14 states in a cross-section of the country. Looking at variables such as gender, age, and marital status, the researchers found that the majority of participants believed that witnesses come into court expecting to tell the truth. A minority of them believed an inconsistency invalidated the entire testimony, a larger group did not believe one inconsistency would invalidate all of the witness's testimony, and the rest were undecided. However, the latter two groups agreed they would want to look at the totality of the testimony before making a decision (Stuhan et al., 2007). The authors also acknowledged that the participants responded without context and most real-life inconsistencies are more nuanced than overt. Regardless, the experience showed that jury behavior is not predictable, but the services of an experienced forensic psychologist can help deter at least some of the surprise (Gomez, 2013).

Expert Testimony

Prior to presenting the cases that laid the foundation for expert testimony in American courts, further information about the presentation of testimonial evidence can clarify the issues at hand. As has been stated, whether the case is criminal or civil, it is conducted through the introduction of evidence into the record. Chaos would take over, however, if state and federal courts did not have rules about the evidence that could be admitted in the course of litigation. Since the point of any case is to get to the facts to determine the applicable law, the first rule of evidence is that it must be relevant so that it can be used to support the truth of the matter asserted by the parties. That being said, its probative value must outweigh its prejudicial effect (Federal Rule of Evidence 403). In other words, it must be more probative to elicit the ultimate facts for jury deliberation, rather than biased for or against any of the parties.

Although not specifically on point for the admission of expert testimony, an example of a strong prejudicial effect would be the admission of hearsay evidence. This might be the "he said, she said" situation with which almost everyone has some familiarity or the eavesdropping scenario. For example, going back to our pencil case, a witness for the seller attempts to testify that she heard the buyer say to someone that he was sorry he had ordered so many pencils prior to receiving the order. This is hearsay since the buyer did not say it to her, and she may have misunderstood the context. Further, because of the content of the statement, its prejudicial effect would almost certainly outweigh its probative value. The seller would object to the admission of the testimony on the grounds that it was hearsay, and the jury could easily be prejudiced by such a statement and give it too much weight in its decision making. This last risk is a key point, and as the cases will show, is the foundational reason the admission of expert testimony has had such a difficult history.

Competency

In tracing the course of a criminal trial in Chapter 4, the issue of the defendant's competency was raised at several points. The reason competency is mentioned in this chapter is that the problem is always addressed in a civil proceeding when it is raised.

In fact, it is probably considered one of the major issues addressed in mental health law, providing professional opportunities for evaluators, expert witnesses, and researchers (Perlin, Champine, Dlugacz & Connell, 2008). Aside from requiring the services of forensic mental health professionals in conjunction with a criminal proceeding, the forensic psychologist may be asked to evaluate competence to enter into a contract, write a will, consent to medical treatment, or give any type of informed consent, as well as suitability for involuntary commitment (Perlin et al., 2008; *Schloendorff v. Society of New York Hospitals*, 1914).[3]

When the mental health professional is called in to evaluate and/or testify as to competency in any of these circumstances, the first task is to operationalize the referral question or, as presented in Chapter 3, put the problem into context and determine the standard for competence in the particular situation. Is it the competence to sign a contract, stand trial, or write a will? In each situation, the facts will be different, and the standard might be as well (Perlin et al., 2008). It is not, however, the role of the evaluator to make the actual determination of competence. For each situation, that is a legal question, and the answer will be based on the psychological evaluation.

Malingering

Although malingering is not a mental disorder according to *the Diagnostic and Statistical Manual of Mental Disorders*, fifth edition (*DSM-5*; American Psychiatric Association, 2013), it is listed as another "condition that may be a focus of clinical attention" and diagnosing it may often require the services of a mental health professional (American Psychiatric Association, 2013, p. 726). Malingering is a purposeful behavior of producing "false or grossly exaggerated physical or psychological symptoms, motivated by external incentives" and should be strongly suspected if (among other things) the "context of the presentation" is medicolegal such as referred by "an attorney . . . for examination, or the individual self-refers while litigation or criminal charges are pending" (*DSM-5*, 2013, pp.726–727).

Assessing for malingering is fundamental to forensic evaluations, and several standardized instruments are available to aid the clinician (Vitacco, Rogers, Gabel, & Munizza, 2007). By 2010, there were 60,000 annual requests to evaluate defendants for competence to stand trial, which made it by far the most often requested forensic evaluation (Soliman & Resnick, 2010). The evaluator's job in this instance is not only to determine whether the individual knows enough about the nature of the case as to be able to assist in his or her own defense, but also to cut through any feigning of symptoms (Soliman & Resnick, 2010). As was seen in Table 3.1, a forensic interview needs to be approached with a certain amount of cynicism. The mental health professional not only has the interview, standardized instruments, and background information available for this purpose, but also has clinical experience and expertise on which to rely.

This last factor, clinical experience, may be the most dependable tool for the forensic interview. Whether the subject is looking for personal or financial gain, avoiding incarceration, or possibly just seeking a sympathetic listener, the experienced forensic psychologist knows before the interview begins exactly what to look for (Vitacco et al., 2007; also see Chapter 3 for Dr. James Earnest's interview). Several years ago, a clinician and I were the panelists for a doctoral student's first oral comprehensive examination. The client was a woman who was living in a shelter with her children as she and her estranged husband were arguing over the terms of a divorce and custody of their children. As the student ably and thoroughly made her way through the client's story of domestic violence, childhood abuse, and living in a shelter, something about the story just did not ring true. After the completion of the presentation, we began asking the student questions about her time with the client. My colleague's vast amount of clinical experience in forensic settings quickly brought out what the student had not seen: There was definitely the possibility of malingering in the client's story.: The father was seeing his children and bringing them back on time, allegations of her own child abuse were vague and inconsistent, and she never seemed to be able to give a reason for living in a shelter. Unfortunately, students do not usually have an opportunity to follow through with an individual client, but my colleague and I are quite comfortable that this student never again let the possibility of malingering escape her inquiries.

SPOTLIGHT ON CASES

For Background of Psychologists' Expert Testimony

Although the standard for admitting expert testimony had been determined almost 40 years earlier and would be revised 30 years later, psychologists were not allowed to testify as experts until *Jenkins v. United States* was decided in 1962.

Jenkins v. United States (1962)

Facts: In 1959, Vincent Jenkins was arrested and indicted for several felonies. Due to his defense of insanity, he was committed to a psychiatric facility to determine his competency to stand trial and his mental condition at the time of the commission of the crime. Because so many doctors and test results ensued for more than a year, the results of the findings of the mental health professionals are presented as a timeline with the doctors who evaluated and diagnosed. All information is directly from the United States (U.S.) Supreme Court case:

1. October 20 and 22, 1959: Dr. L, the chief psychologist supervised the administration of tests and Jenkins was interviewed by a psychiatrist, Dr. S. His IQ score was 63, which at that time was labeled as "high moron." The psychiatrist diagnosed him as having a "mental defect."

2. November 25, 1959: These findings were confirmed by another psychiatrist, Dr. Mc, and Jenkins was judged incompetent to stand trial.

3. February 25 and March 2, 1960: Another psychologist, Dr. T,. found Jenkins' IQ to be 74, a borderline IQ score, but diagnosed him with schizophrenia.

4. October 3, 1960: Dr. O interviewed Jenkins; Dr. C, a psychiatrist, reviewed Dr. O's test reports and could not find any evidence of mental disease.

5. After October 3, 1960: Dr. I, then chief psychologist, reviewed Dr. T's findings (see point 3) and Jenkins' past history and

administered one part of a six-part test; Dr. I agreed with Dr. T. that Jenkins had schizophrenia.

6. November 6, 1960: After notification that he was not suffering from mental disease or deficiency, Vincent Jenkins was found competent to stand trial.

7. Prior to trial: Drs. S and Mc, two psychiatrists, asked Dr. L, the first psychologist, to retest the defendant. This time his IQ was 90, within an average range, and the psychiatrists revised their diagnoses to be schizophrenia, a psychosis, without reexamining him.

Procedural History: The federal district court, on its own motion (sua sponte), excluded Drs. S and Mc's revised diagnoses because the report came from a psychologist. Jenkins was convicted at trial and appealed the conviction. The trial court excluded the diagnosis as a matter of law rather than allowing the jury to make the determination. The defendant appealed the jury verdict to the D.C. Circuit Court of Appeals.

Issue: Given that psychologists administer assessments, should that evidence be admissible as expert testimony?

Holding: Since psychiatrists do not administer or interpret psychological tests, it is well known that in the normal course of practicing their profession, psychiatrists rely on the reports of psychologists. The lack of medical training does not in and of itself exclude a psychologist's expertise. The trial judge erred by automatically excluding the testimony of the psychologists, and admissibility should be based on the qualifications of individual psychologists. The jury then, as trier of fact, can determine how much weight to give the testimony of the psychologist.

Judgment: Reversed and remanded in favor of the appellant, Vincent Jenkins.

Sidebar: Prior to the oral arguments in this case, two Amicus Curiae briefs were filed: One was in support of the admission of psychological expert testimony, and the other was opposed to it (*Jenkins v. United States*, 1962). Not surprisingly, the former was filed by the American Psychological Association; the latter was filed by the American Psychiatric Association. The former's brief defined psychology as the scientific study of human behavior and delved deeply into its scientific history by raising the work of Wilhelm Wundt in his experimental psychology laboratory in Germany. Wundt, in fact, was the mentor and advisor of James McKeen Cattell (Boring, 1950). The brief went on to talk about the then 20-division American Psychological Association and the stringent rules it observed when allowing in new fellows, members, and associates (Brief, 1962).

Whether Mr. Jenkins was retried or found competent to stand trial was, unfortunately, not reported. The fact is that his case paved the way for psychologists to testify as expert witnesses when the circumstances permit. However, prior to and after the decision in *Jenkins v. United States* (1962), expert testimony was restricted in admissibility for reasons that were only alluded to in Jenkins.

For Admissibility of Expert Testimony

Just as a reminder: All relevant evidence is admissible unless its prejudicial effect outweighs its probative value (Federal Rule of Evidence 403).

Frye v. United States (1923)

Facts: The only facts of record for the case are that Mr. Frye was convicted of second-degree murder. Before and during his trial, his attorney tried to have evidence of lie detector results admitted through the testimony of an expert in the field. The attorney even offered to have Mr. Frye retested in front of the jury. The instrument was called a "systolic blood pressure deception test" and was based on the theory that systolic blood pressure would rise when the subject is trying to deceive and remain stable when responses are truthful (para. 7).

Procedure: The case was tried in the D.C. District Court and appealed to the D.C. Circuit Court of Appeals, the same court Vincent Jenkins would appeal to 39 years later.

Issue: Expert testimony is admissible when the topic is one that lay people would not normally be able to understand without expert instruction. However, science that is in experimental stages may be more confusing than informative for the jury. What is the standard for admission of expert testimony when the science is unfamiliar to most?

Holding: For evidence to be admitted as expert testimony, it needs to have gained general acceptance in the discipline to which it belongs. This deception testing instrument has not gained scientific recognition, and therefore it does not have general acceptance in the scientific community.

Judgment: Lower court is affirmed.

Epilogue: As will be seen in more detail in Chapter 9, deception detection has not come very far in almost a century. No lie detector instrument has as yet been invented that is considered scientifically sound enough that its results can be admitted into court.

The *Frye* rule or **general acceptance test** became and remained the standard for admission of expert testimony in federal and most, if not all, state courts for the next 70 years, even though the case had never reached the U.S. Supreme Court. In 1993, a U.S. Supreme Court case that was originally civil rather than criminal, and that never even got to the trial stage, replaced the *Frye* rule in federal courts and in most state courts as well (Morgenstern, 2017).

Daubert et al. v. Merrell Dow Pharmaceuticals, Inc. (1993)

Facts: The plaintiffs are parents and their children who were born with "serious birth defects" (para. 2). The mothers of these children had taken the drug Bendectin, which was manufactured by the defendant, during their pregnancies. The plaintiffs have evidence of studies that show a link between the drug and the birth defects.

Procedural History: The plaintiffs filed their suit in California Superior Court based on a product liability claim (negligence in manufacturing). The defendant had the case removed[4] to federal district court based on diversity jurisdiction. Prior to trial, the defendant moved for summary judgment. This motion basically states that there is no arguable issue of fact for trial and is rarely granted. However, here the defendant presented evidence that no published studies had shown the drug to cause birth defects. The plaintiffs attempted to counter by presenting their own expert evidence of various types of studies that showed a possible link. Both the trial court and the Ninth Circuit Court of Appeals rejected the plaintiff's evidence as not being generally accepted in the scientific community.

It had not been published, no statistical significance was shown, and it was not subjected to peer review.

Issue: Has the general acceptance test been superseded by the Federal Rules of Evidence?

Holding: There is now a federal rule that obviates the reason for the *Frye* rule in federal courts. Federal Rule of Evidence 702 basically states that expert testimony should be admitted if that testimony will help the trier of fact. To ensure that a prejudicial effect will not outweigh the probative value of the testimony, the expert must be qualified by knowledge, skill, experience, training, and/or education. The testimony must be the product of reliable principles and methods. Further, because of the potential for prejudice, the judge now has discretion in admitting this expert testimony.

Judgment: Reversed and remanded.

Epilogue: In 1995, the Ninth Circuit Court of Appeals reheard the plaintiffs' claim observing the new standard for admissibility of expert testimony (*Daubert v. Merrell Dow Pharmaceuticals, Inc.* [on remand]). At this time, all the proffered plaintiff expert evidence was reviewed by the appeals court, which came to the same conclusion under the Daubert standard that it had under the *Frye* rule. The evidence presented was not obtained through a reliable and valid scientific method, and the only expert willing to testify could say no more than the drug could cause birth defects. So, although the case had set a new standard for admissibility of expert testimony, the plaintiffs lost.

For Malingering

Romano v. Steelcase (2010)

Facts: Kathleen Romano sued Steelcase for injuries suffered when she fell from what she claimed was a defective chair in her office. Steelcase manufactured the chair, and Educational and Institutional Cooperative Services distributed it. Romano claimed her injuries required several surgeries and were permanent, leaving her with restricted movement. To prepare a defense, Steelcase's attorneys asked for and then subpoenaed the private information Romano posted on her social media sites. Apparently what they had seen on the public posts gave them reason to believe that the private posts would reveal that the plaintiff's injuries were not as severe as she claimed. Plaintiff Romano refused to allow the access.

Procedure: Kathleen Romano filed a personal injury action against Steelcase and Educational and Institutional Cooperative Services in the Supreme Court (state trial court) in New York.

This case had not yet gone to trial when the defendants moved to compel consent to see plaintiff's private social media pages. The plaintiff invoked the Stored Communications Act of 1986, which prohibits such social media entities from disclosing information without the consent of the account holder.

Issue: For the legal purpose of this case, the issue is about the plaintiff's right to privacy. However, the cautionary tale for our purposes is about how important a finding of malingering might be in a civil case and how social media can influence that finding.

Rule: Because the postings on social media sites had already been made public and the sites caution users/members that they post at their own risk, any expectation of privacy was deemed not reasonable. Further, New York has a state law requiring full disclosure from both sides of litigation of "all non-privileged matter which is material and necessary to the defense or prosecution of an action" (CPLR §3101). The plaintiff's social network profiles were necessary and material to the defense, and what was available on the public page made it reasonable for the defendant to want to see the rest of it.

Judgment: The court ordered that defendants be given access to all of the plaintiff's past, present, and deleted social media entries.

Caution: Although there is no information regarding the outcome of Ms. Romano's case, it must be assumed that even if she proved her liability case, the damage portion must have been significantly reduced from her original plea. If the defendants found what they expected, they uncovered an excellent example of malingering for personal gain.

A New Tort

As has been repeated throughout these chapters, the forensic psychologist must have familiarity with and understanding of the law and the legal system. In 1968, the Supreme Court of California made new law when it recognized the tort of **negligent infliction of emotional distress** (*Dillon v. Legg*, 1968; Nolan & Ursin, 1981). The very term "emotional distress," without accompanying physical harm, connotes work for the mental health professional and the need to understand both the emotional and legal issues for what could be a rather nebulous diagnosis and cause of action (Day & Hall, 2016).

To begin with, negligent torts are different from intentional torts, in that the elements are very specific and must be proven by a preponderance of the evidence according to the facts. To recover damages in a negligence case, the plaintiff must show that the defendant owed a duty to the plaintiff that was breached, and the breach of that duty was the actual and proximate cause of damage to the plaintiff. Recovering damages in negligence actions is different from the standard in intentional torts, in that the plaintiff must show actual compensable damage (*Dillon v. Legg*, 1968).

Dillon v. Legg (1968)

Facts: The defendant, Legg, hit and killed the plaintiff's daughter while she was crossing a road. This part of Dillon's action was based on the fact that she witnessed the negligent action of Legg, and suffered from mental and physical pain as a result. The plaintiff's other daughter was also close enough to see the collision and was caused physical and mental pain as well.

Procedure: Legg answered Dillon's complaint with a motion for judgment on the pleadings based on previous law that stated there was no duty owed to the plaintiff unless she could show she feared for her own safety—namely, because she was in a "zone of danger." The trial court granted that motion but denied the defendant's motion for summary judgment based on the sister's claim. There was a possibility the facts would show the sister was within the "zone of danger" at the time.

Issue: Does a defendant owe a duty to a plaintiff who was out of the zone of danger when the negligent act took place?

Holding: The defendant owes a duty to every foreseeable victim in a negligence action. Here, it is foreseeable the mother who watched her child get hit by a car would suffer harm. The test will be whether an ordinary individual, the defendant, should have reasonably foreseen the risk of harm to a third person, regardless of whether the person was in a zone of danger. Imposing a zone of danger on circumstances such as this is artificial and arbitrary. However, decisions about applications should be made on a case-by-case basis.

Judgment: Reversed for the plaintiff.

Dissent: The dissent was based on two principles: There would be a flood of litigation based on claims of emotional distress, and many of those would be false claims (malingering).

FOCUS ON CAREERS

Dr. Jay Finkelman is a nationally recognized expert witness who has testified equally on behalf of plaintiffs and defendants since the 1970s. He has an MBA and received his PhD from New York University. Dr. Finkelman also has an MLS (Master of Legal Studies) and is a fellow of the American Psychological Association, the prestigious American Association of Forensic Psychologists (AAFP), and the American Board of Professional Psychologists (ABPP), among other professional organizations. Dr. Finkelman's PhD is in industrial/organization psychology, and although he has been asked to testify as an expert in criminal cases, he reserves his expertise for civil matters such as workplace issues including wrongful termination, sexual harassment, conflicts of interest, and human resources management.

Dr. Finkelman is and has been an academician who maintains a professorship and department chairmanship in a postgraduate industrial/organization program. He says that teaching, researching, and presenting give him not only great personal and professional satisfaction, but also much credibility when called upon for his expert testimony. His expertise is well known among the business law firms that have been employing and recommending his services for several decades. To date, he has testified in 58 trials for an equal number of plaintiffs and defendants,

(*continued*)

(*continued*)

and has sat for numerous depositions, declarations, and other forms of evidence for attorneys' use in trial and negotiations. As described in other parts of this chapter, the admission of his testimony as an expert has been challenged based on the "*Daubert* standard,*"* and the scope of his testimony can be and is limited by the court. As with the testimony of experts in all scientific areas, Dr. Finkelman needs to be aware of and careful not to voice legal opinions.

In fact, Dr. Finkelman's expert testimony was the subject of an appeal by the University of California as defendant in a wrongful termination case (*Kotla v. Regents of University of California*, 2004). The plaintiff, Dee Kotla, sued the defendant for wrongful termination as a retaliatory gesture, which. if correct, violates the Fair Employment and Housing Act (FEHA) (*Kotla v. Regents of University of California*, 2004). Dr. Finkelman's expertise in human resources satisfied the trial judge and, over the defense's objections, he was allowed to testify that the particular facts of the case were indications or evidence of retaliation, as the plaintiff asserted. The jury returned a verdict for the plaintiff of approximately $1 million. The defendant appealed on the grounds that the expert's testimony should never have been admitted and that once admitted, it exceeded the scope of allowable expert testimony. Even though the trial court had not allowed Dr. Finkelman to testify as to the ultimate facts, what was allowed prejudiced the jury to give his testimony too much weight.

The appeals court agreed with the defendant, and reversed for the University of California. However, in doing so, the court also made it clear that experts such as Dr. Finkelman would and should be allowed to testify as to human resources management. The court rejected the defendant's claim that human resources was not valid and stated, "testimony on predicate issues within the expertise of a human resources expert is clearly permissible" (*Kotla v. Regents of the University of California*, 2014, fn. 6). When

(*continued*)

(*continued*)

the case was retried in 2005, Dr. Finkelman was again employed as an expert. One assumes his testimony for this trial was limited in scope, and the jury more than tripled the plaintiff's original award to $5.9 million (Nielsen, 2005).

Ten years later, the University of California, this time the Los Angeles campus (UCLA), was again sued by an employee (Terhune, 2014). Dr. Robert Pedowitz claimed that one year after his hiring, he had been demoted from being a department chair because he had reported physician violations and conflicts of interest among medical personnel. UCLA claimed he was demoted due to poor leadership abilities. While these facts certainly explain why Dr. Finkelman's expertise might be required during such a case, what makes this case interesting is that Dr. Finkelman was employed by the defendant, the University of California. The case was settled prior to a jury verdict, so the impact of Dr. Finkelman's testimony remains unknown (J. Finkelman, personal communication, April 3, 2017; Terhune, 2017).

IN THE NEWS

On June 23, 2017, *The Wall Street Journal* reported a rather unusual use for the polygraph test. Phil Heasley won $2,818,662 in a fishing tournament for catching a 76.5-pound marlin. As is the established tournament's custom, Heasley, who had paid $1,000 to enter the tournament, was required to take a lie detector test. Both he and the captain of the boat he was on failed the test—not once, but twice. Because the organizers wanted to redistribute the winnings, the matter ended up in federal court, where the judge found not just that the parties were deceptive about violating tournament rules on their lie detector tests. but violated other tournament rules as well. The "defense had relied heavily on discrediting the accuracy of lie detector tests" (Clarke, 2017, p. A9). The attorney for Heasley stated that courts do not allow in polygraph results as evidence because they are subjective and only 50% accurate.

SUMMARY

This chapter addressed the forensic psychologist's role in civil cases. Evidence, its admissibility, and the weight given to it set the scene for a series of cases that followed. A timeline of sorts was established to present cases that directly affect the role of psychologists in court: *Jenkins v. United* States (1962), *Frye v. United States* (1923), and *Daubert v. Merrell Dow Pharmaceuticals* (1993) all address expert testimony. Other topics in civil law were illustrated through considering additional cases. *Romano v. Steelcase* (2010) was used to explain malingering and the impact of social media on the courts. Prior to the development of social media, the facts of *Dillon v. Legg* (1968) were responsible for the creation of a new tort: negligent infliction of emotional distress. The career of Dr. Jay Finkelman was the focus of the interview for this chapter, as he described his work as an expert witness in civil matters. Finally, the experience of Phil Heasley was the topic of the "In the News" feature. Heasley had failed a lie detector test twice after supposedly catching a prize-winning fish. Although lie detector evidence is not considered accurate enough to be admissible in a court of law, Heasley's failure was enough for him to be stripped of his winnings.

DISCUSSION QUESTIONS

1. As mentioned, malingering does not occur just in criminal cases or even forensic settings. What are some other reasons why individuals might malinger? Does personal gain necessarily mean harm to another?

2. The subject matter of the appeal of *Frye v. United States* (1923) is the admissibility of lie detector evidence. Deception detection is an important part of the work of the forensic psychologist, and the topic is heavily researched by academics, students, and medical professionals. Yet, almost 100 years later, lie detection evidence remains inadmissible in every court in the United States. Why do you think this is?

3. In reading the facts of and discussion about *Dillon v. Legg* (1968), what are your thoughts about the dissent's concern for

the potential of malingering with the recognition of the new tort of negligent infliction of emotional distress? Why would the services of a forensic psychologist be valuable in such a case?

NOTES

1. Even if the defendant is being tried on a criminal matter, if competency is at issue, it is a civil matter; see Chapter 4 for further information.
2. Most of the published research regarding eyewitness testimony (e.g., accuracy, confidence) has been conducted regarding criminal matters, as in perpetrator identification. However, the same challenges would apply in civil matters.
3. Aside from the reference in this chapter, for further reading on competency in legal matters, attorney Michael L. Perlin is a recognized expert on mental disability law. He is a law professor and prolific author who has written over 30 books and published numerous articles. Among his titles are *Mental Disability Law* (3 volumes), *Law and Mental Disability* (1994), *Mental Disability and the Death Penalty* (2013), and *Mental Disability Law: Cases and Materials* (2005).
4. Removal is an option available to the parties when the state and federal courts have simultaneous jurisdiction over a case. Here, the defendant must have thought its chances of winning in federal court were better than in state court. Federal jurisdiction here was based on diversity, meaning no plaintiffs resided in the same state as the defendant (28 USC 1332).

REFERENCES

American Bar Association. (2002). *ABA model rules of professional conduct.* Retrieved from https://www.law.cornell.edu/ethics/aba

American Psychiatric Association. (2013). *Diagnostic and statistical manual of mental disorders* (5th ed.). Washington, DC: Author.

American Psychological Association. (2017). *Ethical principles of psychologists and code of conduct.* Washington, DC: Author. Retrieved from http://www.apa.org/ethics/code/ethics-code-2017.pdf

American Psychological Association. (2013). Specialty guidelines for forensic psychology. *American Psychologist, 68*(1), 7–19. doi:10.1037/a0029889

Aronson, E. (2012). *The social animal* (11th ed.). New York, NY: Worth.

Ayres, B. D. Jr. (1997, February 5). Civil jury finds Simpson liable in pair of killings. *New York Times*. Retrieved from http://www.nytimes.com/1997/02/05/us/civil-jury-finds-simpson-liable-in-pair-of-killings.html

Boring, E. G. (1950). *A history of experimental psychology* (2nd ed.). Englewood Cliffs, NJ: Prentice-Hall.

Brief for American Psychological Association as Amicus Curiae Supporting Petitioner. *Jenkins v. United States* 307 F.2d 637 (1962).

California Rules of Professional Conduct. (2017). State Bar of California. Retrieved from http://www.calbar.ca.gov/Attorneys/Conduct-Discipline/Rules/Rules-of-Professional-Conduct/Current-Rules

Clarke, J. (2017, June 23). Congratulations, here's your fishing prize! Now for the Polygraph. *Wall Street Journal*, A1, A9.

Daubert v. Merrell Dow Pharmaceuticals 509 U.S. 579 (1993).

Daubert v. Merrell Dow Pharmaceuticals 43 F.3d 1311 (9th Cir. 1995).

Day, T. R., & Hall, R. C. W. (2016). PTSD and tort law. In C. R. Martin, V. R. Preedy, & V. B. Patel (Eds.), *Comprehensive guide to post-traumatic stress disorders* (pp. 231–244, Abstract). New York, NY: Springer.

Dillon v. Legg 68 Cal. 2d. 728 (1968).

Federal Rules of Evidence 401–403, 702 (1973).

Frye v. United States 293 F. 1013 (1923).

Gomez, M. M. (2013). Setting the right foundation for your witness testimony. *The Legal Intelligencer Blog*. Retrieved from http://thelegalintelligencer.typepad.com/tli/melissa-m-gomez

Grodsky, A. B. (2012, April). Preparing witnesses. *California Lawyer*, 17.

Ito, L. (1995). 9/95 Jury instructions in O.J.'s criminal case. *'Lectric Law Library*. Retrieved from http://www.lectlaw.com/files/cas62.htm

Jenkins v. United States 307 F.2d 637 (1962).

Kotla v. Regents of the University of California 115 /cak, /aoo, 4th 283 (2004).

Leippe, M. R. Eisenstadt, D., Rauch, S. M., & Seib, H. M. (2004). Timing of eyewitness expert testimony, jurors' need for cognition, and case strength as determinant of trial verdicts. *Journal of Applied Psychology*, 89(3), 524–541.

Morgenstern, M. (2017). Daubert v. Frye: A state-by-state comparison. *The Expert Institute*. Retrieved from https://www.theexpertinstitute.com/daubert-v-frye-a-state-by-state-comparison/

Nielsen, J. C. (2005). Human resources management comes of age in the courtroom: California formally enshrines the importance of human resources expert testimony for employment litigation. *Psychologist-Manager Journal*, 8(2), 157–164.

Nolan, V. E. (1981). Negligent infliction of emotional distress: Coherence emerging from chaos. *Hastings Law Journal*, *33*, 583–621.

Perlin, M. L., Champine, P., Dlugacz, H. A., & Connell, M. (2008). *Competence in the law: From legal theory to clinical application*. Hoboken, NJ: Wiley & Sons.

Romano v. Steelcase Inc. 2006-2233 (N.Y. Super. Sept. 21, 2010).

Schloendorff v. Society of New York Hospitals 105 N.E. 92 (N.Y. 1914).

Schweitzer, N. J., & Saks, M. J. (2009). The gatekeeper effect: The impact of judges' admissibility decisions on the persuasiveness of expert testimony. *Psychology, Public Policy, & Law, 15*(1), 1–18.

Simon, S. (1997, January 29). Simpson case jurors begin deliberations. *Los Angeles Times*. Retrieved from http://articles.latimes.com/1997-01-29/news/mn-23251_1_simpson-case

Soliman, S., & Resnick, P. J. (2010). Feigning in adjudicative competency evaluations. *Behavioral Sciences & the Law, 28*, 614–629.

Stuhan, R. G., Gomez, M. M., & Wolfe, D. (2007). Impeaching with prior inconsistent statements. *For the Defense*, 14–21. Retrieved from http://mmgjury.com/publications/mmg/Impeaching_with_Prior_Inconsistent_Statements.pdf

Terhune, C. (2014, April 22). UC oks paying surgeon $10 million in whistleblower-retaliation case. *Los Angeles Times*. Retrieved from http://www.latimes.com/business/la-fi-ucla-doctor-conflicts-20140423-story.html

Uniform Commercial Code, Article 1 General Provisions §1-303 (2001). Retrieved from https://www.law.cornell.edu/ucc/1/1-303

Vitacco, M. J., Rogers, R., Gabel, J., & Munizza, J. (2007). An evaluation of malingering screens with competency to stand trial patients: A known-groups comparison. *Law & Human Behavior, 31*, 249–260.

Wixted, J. T., & Wells, G. L. (2017). The relationship between eyewitness confidence and identification accuracy: A new synthesis. *Psychological Science in the Public Interest, 18*(1), 10–65.

The Forensic Psychologist's Role in Family Court

OVERVIEW

Just as no one book can hope to cover all the subtopics included in forensic psychology, no one chapter can possibly cover all the psycholegal topics inherent in discussing family matters. At the outset, it should be recognized that, with the changing make-up of the American family, this chapter could have been titled "What Is a Family?" Both the law and the study of psychology have necessarily undergone dramatic changes since the turn of the 21st century, although it bears repeating that the law has taken a while to catch up with psychology. Two points must be made when discussing the family. First, psychology and the law, and even biology, often conflict and need time to catch up with each other. Second, to fully understand the depth and breadth of the changes, family matters must be seen from a historical perspective. Those just beginning to develop their interest or starting their careers may wonder what all the drama is about without the background.

The new issues include those raised by **same-sex marriage**, **divorce, transgender** situations, and **child custody**. While some of these are completely new problems, child custody matters are neither new nor particularly straightforward. The state's role with regard to children has always been that the state will act in the **best interest of the children** who come within its jurisdiction. What has changed is what the state thinks is in the best interest of the children. Following child custody awards through several decades will illuminate how that definition has changed. This chapter also explains the multilayered approach the law demands in conducting child custody evaluations and the organizations, courts, and individuals who conduct them. Fitness for **surrogacy, divorce counseling, domestic violence**, and **competency regarding estate issues** are also part of the forensic psychologist's role in family court.

Another topic that is touched upon in this chapter is **suicide**, which is an important research topic for forensic psychologists. The rate of youth suicide is a major social issue as well as a family problem, and the suicide of a family member often destroys the family dynamic (*Teen suicide*, 2013). Further, in an ongoing effort to find motivations, explore the impact of social media (see Chapter 4), and possibly find ways to prevent suicide, a specific role for the forensic psychologist might be to conduct a **psychological autopsy**, which would entail delving into family history and interviewing family members if at all possible.

The cases used to illustrate some of the points of this chapter range over a period of decades to show changes in family structure, both in the psychological sense and in the laws involved. So, although the separation of the legal concerns from the psychological and societal issues is not always clear cut, specific topics addressed include the evolution of marriage laws and attitudes, estate issues within the family, divorce, children, domestic violence, and suicide and the psychological autopsy.

HOW IT WORKS

Background

Keeping in mind that every state makes its own laws regarding families, what follows is meant to give an overview of the evolution of the definition of family, specifically marriage, and the work of the forensic psychologist when the courts become involved. Families are not static in their make-up or relationships. They are often diverse in race, religion, culture, and sexual and gender preference. Therefore, the family issues chosen for elaboration are those that have some relationship to court practice, even if there is not a specific case to cite. In all instances, however, tracing the history of the topic through the cases that are available helps to make sense of the construct. This is also an area that has undergone so much change over the last few years that one cannot help but wonder what the future holds.

Marriage

Under the best of conditions, family issues are filled with emotion and little objectivity. A brief history of marriage in the United States as seen through the laws of one state might help shed some light on the work mental health professionals have done and will continue to do to promote and protect the family (see, for example, *In re Marriage Cases* Amicus Curiae brief, 2008). California's marital law history includes all the relevant issues that law and psychology have been sorting out for at least the last several decades. Nevertheless, it might surprise some to know how recently the legal controversies were actually put to rest. Whether a particular state history is exactly the same does not really matter at this point; legal results are finally consistent throughout the country. What does matter is that the forensic psychologist knows and understands the law and can work within it according to the facts that brought him or her the problem. Remembering that the forensic psychologist is objective, gaining an understanding of the past should provide for more insight into the present. If objectivity is a problem, this is not the area of forensic psychology in which to practice.

Although marriage is a subject that dates back to early Greek civilization, much of this country's family law was based on biblical tradition (Brake, 2016; *In re Marriage Cases*, 2008). In keeping with that tradition, many states defined marriage as a civil union between a man and a woman for the purpose of procreation (Brake, 2016). California, however, even in its initial definition did not use a biblical reference, but took its definition from what was in effect in New York in 1872 (*In re Marriage Cases*, 2008). California defined marriage as a civil contract between a man and a woman who were competent to enter into the contract. Competence was defined by the age of the parties.[1] The contractual nature of marriage has always been recognized, and, therefore, marriage can exist only between parties who have the capacity to contract. As the decades passed, the age of majority or consent changed for various purposes, and finally when the Twenty-Sixth Amendment to the United States (U.S.) Constitution passed in 1971 giving 18-year-olds the right to vote, that became the recognized age of majority for marriage purposes.

Through the years, laws and cases affecting marriage slowly changed the institution. As discussed in Chapter 2, the case of *Griswold v. Connecticut* in 1965 established a marital right to privacy from government interference, although state laws varied as to who was considered validly married. The question became whether a marriage that was valid in one state would be recognized in another state (Grossman, 2015). Generally, states did recognize valid marriages from other states in the interest of promoting family responsibility and stability and facilitating interstate travel (Grossman, 2015). However, if the marriage so offended the public policy of the state that had a stronger relationship with the union, that state did not need to recognize it (Swisher, Miller, & Shapo, 2012).[2]

It is difficult to imagine such a situation occurring today, but the recent movie *Loving* depicted the true story of an interracial couple whose marriage so offended the laws of the state of Virginia that they were given the choice of a felony conviction or leaving the state in 1958 (Buirski & Nichols, 2016; *Loving v. Virginia*, 1967). The Lovings left the state for 5 years, but appealed the case through the courts of Virginia until the United States (U.S.) Supreme Court agreed to rule on the validity of the Virginia miscegenation laws. In a unanimous decision, the Court found the state's argument that the law did not violate equal protection or due process guaranteed by the Fourteenth Amendment was weak. While it applied equally to whites intermarrying as to the people of color who married them, it did not apply to people of color marrying each other. The Court further rejected the argument that the state had an interest in keeping the races separate as having no purpose other than racial discrimination (*Loving v. Virginia*, 1967). At the time, 16 states still had laws barring interracial marriage, and all of the laws became unconstitutional (Grossman, 2015).[3]

While states did begin liberalizing marriage laws and receding from infringing on the privacy of marriage by 1965 owing to the *Griswold v. Connecticut* decision, it was not until 2003 that a state recognized the right of homosexual couples to marry. In *Goodridge v. Massachusetts Department of Public Health*, the Massachusetts state Supreme Court used the *Loving* reasoning that marriage was a fundamental right to conclude that the state constitution provided for same-sex marriage. By 2004, the mayor of San Francisco was performing same-sex marriages in response to the Massachusetts decision but in opposition to California law (Stout, 2004).

The documented stigma of homosexuality dates back to at least 1952, when homosexuality was classified as a mental disorder in the first edition of the *Diagnostic and Statistical Manual of Mental Disorders* (*DSM*) (Brief, 2008). However, by 1973, the *DSM* no longer included homosexuality, as no research had ever provided credible evidence that homosexuality was a disorder (Brief, 2008). Yet, in what might be thought of as another instance of the law not keeping up with psychology, states continued to marginalize their gay citizens. Although the California Supreme Court decided in favor of same-sex marriage, the American Psychological Association's Amicus Curiae brief (2008) in support of the couples in the *In re Marriage Cases* (2008) case delineated other moral and societal reasons that individuals and groups voted to ban gay marriage in California only 10 months later, in November 2008.

The constitutionality of Proposition 8, a would-be state constitutional amendment, wound through state and federal courts until 2013, when the U.S. Supreme Court issued its decision in *United States v. Windsor* and refused to make a ruling in the California case. Briefly, the *Windsor* ruling made unconstitutional the federal Defense of Marriage Act (DOMA), which had prevented legally married same-sex couples from participating in federal **estate tax** and other benefits. The ruling not only ordered the Internal Revenue Service to refund over $300,000 that Ms. Windsor had paid when her spouse died, but also left in place a Ninth Circuit ruling that Proposition 8 was unconstitutional. Within 2 days of the ruling, same-sex marriages resumed in California (Lloyd, 2013).[4]

Finally, in 2015, the U.S. Supreme Court consolidated the cases of 30 individuals from four states who claimed their states' anti-same-sex marriage laws violated their Fourteenth Amendment rights to due process and equal protection (*Obergefell v. Hodges*). In a 5–4 decision, Justice Anthony Kennedy wrote for the majority that same-sex couples "ask for equal dignity in the eyes of the law. The Constitution grants them that right" *(Obergefell v. Hodges,* 2015, p. 28).[5] Marriage laws have now either become or are becoming gender neutral in all states (see, for example, California Family Code §§ 300 et seq.)

Divorce

Divorce, unlike marriage, started out as an adversarial process in the United States. When school children learn about the marriages of Henry VIII, they learn as a matter of fact that the king started a new religion in England because his Catholicism did not provide for divorce from his first wife (Fielder, n.d.). Since Henry was head of state and his church, Catherine of Aragon did not have much choice about the divorce. As with most of our laws, divorce came to the then colonies with that English background and favored the man (Malesky, 2012). Religion, state law, and a double standard contributed to the practice for many decades (Grace, 2010). The adversarial system had what was called fault divorce, and men could find more fault than women to get their divorces. By the middle of the 20th century, civil divorces seemed to be more evenly applied, and by 1970, one state enacted no-fault divorce laws (Bird, n.d.). It is interesting that California was the first no-fault state, while New York, the state from which California took its first definition of marriage, was the last in 2010 (Domestic Relations Law [DRL] § 170.7; *In re Marriage Cases,* 2008). Aside from the 40-year span between the no-fault timing, California has abolished all fault reasons for divorce; New York kept six and added no-fault as the seventh (California Family Code §§ 2310-2313; DRL §§170-170.7).

California has gone even further in trying to eliminate the suggestion of divorce being an adversarial proceeding; it has eliminated the term "divorce" in favor of "dissolution of marriage" and does not allow "specific acts of misconduct" to be admitted as evidence (California Family Code § 2335). Another difference between the states is that in California, the parties can bifurcate the proceedings so that financial affairs can be resolved at some point after the dissolution has been granted (§ 2337). Although California has a waiting period after separating, it is not unusual for financial matters to go through the courts for years after the marriage is legally dissolved (M. Fisher, personal communication, July 19, 2017). New York's no-fault law cannot be invoked unless the parties, among other things, have settled their "economic issues" (DRL § 170.7).

Lest the reader think that all opportunity for a psychological evaluation has been eliminated from the California dissolution of marriage, the two no-fault grounds are that "irreconcilable differences" have led to an irretrievable breakdown of the marriage or, alternatively, one of the parties suffers from incurable insanity. This later ground requires medical or psychiatric testimony be presented (California Family Code § 2310 (a) and (b)).

In California, the parties are called petitioner and respondent; in New York, they are plaintiff and defendant, and there is no insanity grounds for divorce in New York. All the other states seem to fall somewhere in between New York and California, both geographically and in their divorce laws. However, whether there is fault or no fault, financial settlement or not, if there are children, there will be issues of custody and visitation.

Children

In this chapter, children are discussed only in the limited context of custody and visitation. However, those are not issues only in dissolution or divorce situations. Child custody issues often arise when a parent dies, in adoption and surrogacy situations, and even regarding stepchildren. Although the law seems clear on most, if not all, of these matters, interpretation and actuality are not always in sync with the laws. At the outset, it must be remembered that the state's duty is to act in the best interest of the child (California Family Code § 3040; Schepard, n.d.). The problem is that even though state laws list what is in the best interest of the child with as much specificity as can be generally interpreted, the terms are not always applicable in any given situation (Schepard, n.d.). So while the child custody evaluator does not make legal decisions, conducting the evaluation is obviously a demanding process.

In 2011, the American Association of Matrimonial Lawyers published Child Custody Evaluation Standards, an aspirational but unenforceable list of goals for the education and behavior of child custody evaluators. These goals and guidelines complement state requirements and provide a necessary framework within which the child custody evaluator works with families, courts, and attorneys.

Custody

Historically, the best interest of a small child, specifically one under 7 years old, was served by giving custody to the mother, unless she was proven to be unfit; this Tender Years Doctrine was abandoned when fathers' rights groups became active and vocal (Schepard, n.d.). Since most family codes are now gender neutral, the preference list is also more neutral (see, for example, California Family Code § 3040 listing order of preference for awarding custody). While states that have joint custody statutes seem to prefer to award custody jointly to parents, the statutes also say that if custody is going to only one parent, consideration needs to be given to the parent who is most likely to allow the other parent frequent contact (California Family Code § 3040). Abuse and lifestyle of the parents need to be taken into consideration, but while poverty of one parent may be a factor, it cannot be determinative of a custody award. Custom, circumstances, location, and even personal experience may play a role in awarding custody. Although *Painter v. Bannister* (1966) was decided over 50 years ago, the standard for a custody award in Iowa was no different from the standard anywhere in the United States today: After reviewing all the evidence, what is in the best interest of the child?

Painter v. Bannister (1966)

Facts: Harold Painter's wife and daughter were killed in an automobile accident in 1962. Shortly thereafter, Harold asked the Bannisters, his in-laws, to care for his then 5-year-old son, Mark. The Bannisters lived in Iowa, where they enjoyed an upper-middle-class lifestyle. Harold had lived in various states on the West Coast and did not have steady employment. The court reported that Mark was undisciplined with no friends when he went to live with his grandparents, but that had changed since. He was happy and had friends. Harold remarried about a year after the Bannisters took Mark to live with them and settled in northern California. He then asked the Bannisters to return Mark, and they refused. By that time, Mark had been living with his grandparents for over 2 years. The facts revealed that the lifestyles of the two families contrasted in religious observance, education, home environment, and politics. The grandparents had been opposed to their daughter's marriage to a man they called a "hippie."

Procedural History: Harold filed for custody of Mark in Iowa. The Iowa trial court, after reviewing all the information and rejecting the testimony of a child psychologist, gave custody to the father. The Bannisters refused to return Mark and appealed to the Iowa Supreme Court. A change of custody was stayed pending the Supreme Court decision.

Issue: In all custody cases, the issue is, what is in the best interest of the child?

Rule: The facts of each case must be weighed according to the applicable law. In Iowa, a preference should be given to the parent; here, the parent is qualified to assume custody. Parental wishes need to be considered; the mother's will nominated Harold Painter as custodian. Professional testimony should be given weight in making the decision; the child psychologist who examined Mark is highly credentialed and concluded custody should remain with the Bannisters.

Holding: Of all the factors to be taken into consideration, stability is what is in the best interest of the child. Mark lived with his grandparents for almost 3 years and looked to them as parental figures, and the child psychologist recommended he continue to live with them.

Judgment: The Iowa Supreme Court reversed the trial court's decision, and custody remained with the Bannisters.

Epilogue: Less than 2 years after the Iowa Supreme Court ruling and a refusal by the U.S. Supreme Court to hear the case, Mark Painter went to permanently live with his father in California (Weisbrod, 2006). The Bannisters did not dispute the move.

The decision in *Painter v. Bannister* (1966) was controversial and highly debated and is still considered a landmark case with far-reaching ramifications (Weisbrod, 2006). What is in the best interest of a child, when all parties are fit, remains problematic for the law, psychology, and all parties. As families change and the rules seem to change as well, the child custody evaluator's job becomes more complex, and the statutory requirements do not tell the whole story. Such evaluators administer psychological and cognitive tests to the parties; synthesize their results; interview the adults, children, and other interested parties; and always keep in mind that their objective clinical judgment should be the strongest guide.

New Rules

California has a rather unusual law that is shared by about 10 other states (Associated Press, 2017). The Family Code in California, as amended in 2014, provides for the possibility that a child might have more than two parents (§3040 (3) (d)), as a result of statute, adoption, or a custody ruling. Advocates say this reflects our modern family (Associated Press, 2017). The courts and experts are divided, however, about the benefits of children having three parents. The "anti" group invokes studies that show two-parent households are more stable and children who are reared in two-parent homes do better educationally and psychologically (Associated Press, 2017). However, this research is not based on three-parent families; as of the end of 2015, while acknowledging dramatic changes in the living arrangements of American families, research on three-parent families seemed nonexistent (*Parenting in America*).

Legally and traditionally, only two types of parents have had rights and obligations regarding children: biological and adoptive. At one time, a woman who gave birth was conclusively presumed to be the mother of the child, and if the child was born during marriage, the husband was presumed to be the father (Smernoff, 1996). The state's unstated interest was in making sure a child had a stable, supportive, and supporting home. Adoption laws terminated biological parental rights and invested them in adoptive parents. When medical science advanced enough that women were being inseminated by donor sperm, laws were enacted to protect the stranger donor from obligations to the children (California Family Code 7613(b)). By the end of the 20th century, women were acting as surrogates for other women who for one reason or another could not become pregnant. Problems arose when women refused to give up the babies they had carried for 9 months after they were born. Although there were contracts between the parties, the courts did not always enforce them. The law stated then and now that contracts to sell babies were and are illegal and void (*In re Matter of Baby M.*, 1988).

Then, medical science advanced so that a surrogate might be inseminated with an embryo that was not biologically hers. Litigation ensued, and decisions were made on a case-by-case basis. Now, several states have enacted surrogacy laws predetermining who the parents are, depending upon the intent of the parties. Many attorneys and psychologists specialize in this type of work, trying to prevent problems before they occur. One psychologist's sole practice is based on attorney referral for fitness for surrogacy. As with any forensic interview, the psychologist acts as an objective evaluator looking for the answers to questions that the laws and the courts would ask (see, for example, California Family Code §7613.5, §7613 (b)). The forms and contracts that result from these arrangements are carefully worded so they cannot be interpreted as contracts for the sale of babies. Some of the statutes even include possible templates for the contracts and caution the parties to seek legal advice (see, for example, California Family Code §§ 7613 et seq.).

Old Problems

The U.S. Supreme Court decision in *Obergefell v. Hodges* (2015) may have finally put to rest the question of same-sex marriage in the United States, but it also brought out the potential for psycholegal issues for children of gay couples if both partners could not share parenting rights. Justice Kennedy related the stories of three of the couples asking the court for relief. A lesbian couple from Michigan had three adopted children. Only one of them could adopt, however, since Michigan law at the time allowed only one parent in a same-sex relationship to adopt. This meant that the nonparent had no legal rights or obligations and could not make medical, educational, or any emergency decisions on behalf of the child.

Adoption is not a new concept, and today an adopted child is treated in the law as if the child is the biological child of the adoptive parents. However, all adopted children came from biological parents, and issues of consent seem to keep reappearing (Consent to Adoption by State, n.d.). At one time, an unmarried mother had sole custody of her child, and only her consent was needed to terminate parental rights. However, that has changed, and the marital status of the parents is immaterial. Further, successful arguments have been made several years after the fact that either the mother was coerced into relinquishing her child or the father did not know about the child and could not give consent. In these instances, child custody evaluators are called in to conduct investigations, assessments, and interviews to help the courts make custody decisions.

Foster parenting is a legal construct that often requires court intervention. Foster parents have no legal claim to the children in their care and receive a stipend for providing that care. Issues of biological parent visitation, petitions to regain custody of their children, and termination of parental rights are not unusual while these children are in foster care. The fitness of the foster parent can also be an issue.

Finally, today's family often consists of children from previous marriages or relationships of one or both adults. These are stepchildren. Legally, neither they nor the nonparental adults with whom they live have obligations or rights, unless the parent's spouse has legally adopted the child. However, if the adult relationship ends, the nonparent often desires a place in the child's life. Remembering at all times that courts act in the best interest of the child, courts will now hear cases of step-parents, grandparents, and other interested parties who have no legal claim but feel their presence in the lives of these children would be in everyone's best interest. While family law attorneys are aware of which states will hear these types of cases, as they vary from state to state and from case to case, the input of an evaluator will almost always be necessary (see, for example, Frank, 2017).

Domestic Violence

In 2015, *The Daily Beast* printed a story in which Ivana Trump, Donald Trump's first wife, said he had raped her during their marriage (Zadrozny & Mak). Whether Donald Trump did or did not rape Ivana

Trump has never been determined, but what is clear is that his attorney, Michael Cohen, inaccurately responded to the accusation when he said a spouse could not rape a spouse. Spousal rape is a crime in every state (see, for example, California Penal Code § 262; Edelman & Katz, 2015). Historically, there was no such thing as domestic violence among married people. As strange as it might sound to some younger readers, once a woman married, she lost her individual identity and was deemed to have consented to her husband's wishes (Edelman & Katz, 2015).

Domestic violence is legally defined as abuse committed against adults or emancipated minors who are former or current spouses, former or current cohabitants, individuals currently or formerly engaged or dating, or individuals having a child in common (California Penal Code § 13700). The abuse can be psychological, physical, or sexual. Specific domestic violence laws vary from state to state, and enforcement varies as well. However, it seems generally agreed that the states have finally recognized the need and enacted the necessary laws to protect the abused and punish and potentially rehabilitate the abuser (*Altafulla v. Ervin*, 2015). Unfortunately, in too many instances the abused spouse denies the abuse, lives in isolation, is afraid to leave, or returns to further abuse (Sachs & Gomberg, 2004, 2009).

Estates

As noted earlier in regard to marriage, capacity is the underlying psychological issue for consideration in family court. *United States v. Windsor* (2013) brought up the legal issue of an estate bequest, a federal tax event, to lay the foundation for the eventual invalidation of that part of DOMA that prohibited giving a tax benefit to a same-sex spouse upon the death of the other spouse. The Supreme Court decision in that case had far-reaching consequences for our society. Most estate cases are much less influential and involve only a small group of family members at most. However, when a bequest is challenged, forensic psychologists may be called upon to offer their expert opinion as to the intent or capacity of the decedent (Gutheil, 2007). Although challenges to testamentary bequests are rare and even more rarely granted, the fact that estate bequests are a topic for forensic psychology make them relevant to this discussion.

The most common reasons for the challenges are lack of capacity and undue influence, and most frequently the challenger is a family member who felt he or she did not get a fair share because the decedent lacked the capacity to understand the consequences of his or her actions. Sometimes the challenger will claim that the person who received the gift had exerted undue influence over the donor (Taylor, 2012).

In a perfect world, individuals would have psychological experts examine their capacity to write a will when they actually write their wills (Perlin, Champine, Dlugacz, & Connell, 2008). Alternatively, they could give their possessions away while they are still alive, and a psychological examination could occur at that time. Unfortunately, that is rarely the case. The only way the expert can determine if testamentary capacity existed is to amass as much data as possible and to have a clear understanding of what testamentary capacity entails (Gutheil, 2007).

California's Probate Code §§ 6100 and 6100.5 (1985) are typical of state laws defining testamentary capacity: First, the individual must be 18 years or older and of sound mind. Section 6100.5 defines sound mind as understanding the nature and extent of his or her property, knowing who the natural heirs would be, understanding the plan the will is making, and not suffering from delusions or hallucinations. The assumption is that the individual was of sound mind at the time of making the will, and that assumption must be rebutted by the challenger (Taylor, 2012). Historically, courts have interpreted this capacity standard to be very low, somewhere below the requisite capacity to contract (Gutheil, 2007; Rushing, 2016). However, in 1995, the California legislature enacted the Due Process in Competence Determinations Act (Rushing, 2016).

According to retired California Judge Elaine Rushing, this Act resulted from the development of psychiatry and psychology requiring the updating of the probate rules for capacity. As she notes, the specificity of the findings required by Probate Code §§ 810–812 put a much larger burden on the challenger and are not lawyer friendly; some "commentators opined they virtually necessitate the use of expert witnesses" (Rushing, 2016, para. 11). Attorneys who write wills, trusts, and complete estate plans usually ask their clients only the basic questions necessary to write the documents and assess the clients through general observation. According to Rushing (2016), the additional code sections have created the burden of judging the complexity of the document and then, if the document is complex, assessing for the client's alertness and attention, information- and thought-processing skills, and ability to modulate mood and affect, as required by Probate Code § 811. It seems as if to some extent, the California legislature either expects estate planning attorneys to act as forensic psychologists or to partner with a forensic psychologist whenever a complex estate plan is at issue. Another option is to employ the forensic psychologist to conduct a psychological autopsy (Canter, 2000). As will be seen, this procedure can be a valuable tool in understanding the decedent's state of mind prior to death.

Suicide and Psychological Autopsy[6]

Historically, suicide and its attempt were illegal, violative of certain religious tenets, and/or excluded from insurance death payments (Lawrence, Oquendo, & Stanley, 2015; Lee, Roser, Ortiz-Ospina, 2016; Rouleau, 2016). Much empirical evidence from worldwide reports has been compiled showing that rates of suicide differ among gender, countries, methods, and age groups and that there are far more suicide attempts each year than are reported (Lee et al., 2016). However, it is generally agreed that whatever statistics have been compiled, for various reasons, they are often inaccurate (Lee et al., 2016; Pappas, 2015). Regardless of motivation, the suicide of a family member causes more problems than the grief any death would cause loved ones. Certain religions refuse to bury a person who committed suicide with a religious ceremony, life insurance policies often have an exclusion for suicide clause, and when the suicide is a child, parents and others feel guilt and confusion. Questions often arise not only as to the why of the suicide, but whether it should become public knowledge. Some may even fear a family trait prompted the suicide.[7] For all these reasons and others not mentioned, finding ways to prevent suicide or at least pinpoint reasons has been a research topic for forensic psychologists and psychiatrists for decades (Luxton, June, & Fairall, 2012).

Suicide

So far in this book suicide has been mentioned at least twice, recalling the deaths of two young people who are thought to have been motivated at least partially by the actions of others. Yet, we do not know what internal motivations there might have been for Tyler Clementi and Conrad Roy III to end their lives. Certainly, the availability of the Internet and other technologies were contributory to the actual acts and are probably contributory to the rise in suicides and suicide attempts in general (Luxton et al., 2012). In 2012, 30,000 individuals in the United States took their own lives, and a substantial number of them were young people (Luxton et al.).

Social media and the Internet are responsible for a new term, "cyberbullying," and estimates of the prevalence of cyberbullying range from 23% of social media users to over 40% (Luxton et al., 2012; Pappas, 2015). Of course, these estimates point to only the newest form of bullying. In 2013, 28% of 12- to 18-year-olds reported being bullied at school. according to the Bureau of Justice Statistics and National Center for Education Statistics Institute of Education Sciences, and schools are reported to be where the majority of bullying takes place (Bullying Statistics and Information, 2017). It should also be kept in mind that these statistics could be underestimates, in that children and adults are often ashamed to admit they have been or feel bullied (Harper, 2013). While bullying is known to be a cause of depression among its victims, and depression is known to be a cause of suicide in both children and adults, much of the time the real cause for the suicide remains unknown (Pappas, 2015).

Psychological Autopsy

The psychological autopsy has existed since 1958 and is a valuable research and clinical tool for use by the forensic psychologist (Snider, Hane, & Berman, 2006). It is not, however, a widely used procedure in the broad field of forensic psychology (Snider et al., 2006). But as suicide rates increase, and as this means of investigation becomes more interesting to forensic psychology student researchers and eventual practitioners, the topic is being included as part of the topic of suicide in general and the added psychological and legal problems for the family.

The forensic aspect is that the circumstances of a death are suspicious and/or the survivors or even law enforcement have a desire to know the exact circumstances surrounding the death (Canter, 2000). The "equivocal death" may need a legal determination for a variety of reasons, including the previously mentioned insurance or just suspicious circumstances. Typically, the cause seems to be suicide, and survivors hope to know the motivation (Canter, 2000; Snider et al., 2006). Psychologically, the family members may be hoping the autopsy will reveal an accidental cause of death (Snider et al., 2006).

A psychological autopsy consists of an accumulation of as many interviews as possible with individuals who were close to the deceased; any medical, work, educational, or other records; and sometimes other professionals to help interpret the findings. This is considered the most direct method for ascertaining the cause(s) of suicide when there is doubt or a question (Cavanaugh, Carson, Sharpe, & Lawrie, 2003; Moskos, Olson, Halbern, Keller, & Gray, 2005). Moskos and colleagues (2005) undertook a study of 151 Utah youths ages 13–21 hoping to find commonalities among their suicides, which occurred over only a 2-year period. Some of the research motivation was due to the high rate of suicide in Utah, which was higher than national rates. What the researchers found at the outset was that of the families they were able to contact (106 families of 151 youths), more than half refused to participate (57, versus 49 agreeing to participate).

While the Moskos et al. (2005) study included enough variables that the researchers did find some commonalities such as mental health issues and at least one person in decedents' lives who recognized some symptoms, the limitations probably made the study ungeneralizable. The families who agreed to be interviewed were the survivors of mostly white male suicides. The nonparticipants were more likely to have been referred to Child Protective Services prior to the suicide. Further, the interviewees were not consistent among the families; some siblings, friends, and other family members did not make themselves available. The researchers also voiced a concern that the grief of losing a loved one and the "stigma associated with mental illness and suicide" could have resulted in "recall bias" on the part of the participants (543). Other researchers have conducted computerized psychological autopsies using archival data to find commonalities among suicides and individually found mental illness and adverse life events to be prominent causes (Cavanaugh et al., 2003; Foster, 2011).

Although these studies and others provided valuable research information and potential avenues for future studies, they also highlight one of the inherent complaints about psychological autopsies (Snider et al., 2006). Psychological autopsies are not standardized and if needed for probate or other reasons will not always stand up to a *Daubert* challenge (see Chapter 5 and Snider et al., 2006). Of course, the *Daubert* standard is required only in federal court, and most probate matters are state issues, but admissibility remains at the discretion of the judge (*Daubert v. Merrell Pharmaceuticals*, 1993). Therefore, because the method can be so valuable, researchers and others are encouraging the standardization of psychological autopsies, presenting another type of challenge for future research (Canter, 2000; Snider et al., 2006).

SPOTLIGHT ON CASES

Although same-sex marriage is now the law of the land, with all the rights, privileges, and obligations that opposite-sex marriage brings, and children in almost one fourth of the states can have three parents, the status of transgender individuals still seems to be somewhat murky in some jurisdictions. With more marriages, there will likely be more divorces with the potential of more child custody problems, and more parents asserting their rights. The changing definition of family will undoubtedly create more work for the forensic psychologist in family court. The illustrative case, while unusual today, may very well be commonplace in the not too distant future. Regardless, there will be work in family court for the forensic psychologist.

In *re the Matter of Thomas T. Beatie v. Nancy J. Beatie* (2014)

Facts: Thomas Beatie was born a female, but knew he was male, and as an adult he went through the requisite 3-year psychological and physical examinations and treatment to become a man. After the procedures were complete, his surgeon signed an affidavit stating that Thomas's true gender had been determined to be male, and he had irreversible surgical procedures as a result. Thomas changed all his legal documents to reflect that he was male, changed his name, and obtained an amended birth certificate stating he was male from his native state of Hawaii. Thomas married Nancy in Hawaii, a state which at the time (2003) only allowed marriages between a man and a woman. Nancy was unable to have children, and Thomas had not yet had his genital surgery. Thomas gave birth during the marriage to three children.

The Beaties moved from Hawaii to Arizona, which also did not validate same-sex marriage. At some time thereafter, Mr. Beatie filed for dissolution of marriage.

Procedural History: When a case is filed, the first thing the court needs to do is determine if it has jurisdiction, the power to make an enforceable decision. In this case, the lower court determined it did not have subject matter jurisdiction, the power to make a decision regarding this marriage. In looking at the facts, particularly the fact that Mr. Beatie had given birth, the court stated it could not render a judgment of dissolution of marriage if a marriage never existed. The reasoning was that the marriage was never valid because it was the marriage of two women; only women can give birth.

Issue: Will Arizona recognize a marriage from another state even if that marriage might not be valid in Arizona?

Rule: A marriage is valid where celebrated if it complies with the legal requirements of that state. If a valid marriage does not offend the policy of the recognizing state, it needs to be recognized.

Holding: Although Mr. Beatie received his amended birth certificate, Arizona is accusing him of having obtained it fraudulently because he did not tell the state he had retained his female genitals. The doctor issued an affidavit stating Mr. Beatie was male, and the doctor knew the facts. Therefore, the marriage was validly entered into in Hawaii as one man and one woman. as it would be in Arizona.

Judgment: The marriage of Thomas and Nancy Beatie was valid in the state of Hawaii, and Arizona has subject matter jurisdiction. Remanded.

FOCUS ON CAREERS

After serving over three decades as a psychologist on the Family Court Panel of one of the largest counties in the United States, **Dr. Clive Kennedy** is a forensic psychologist by experience. He has conducted all forms of family court evaluations as a private and court-appointed evaluator. To qualify to be listed on the directory provided to the courts, attorneys, and private parties, Dr. Kennedy needed to have certain education and experience required by state law. Although the law does not require child custody evaluators to have a doctoral-level education, Dr. Kennedy has a PhD and is a licensed clinical psychologist. Being a licensed mental health professional for at least 5 years is the first requirement for inclusion. Among Dr. Kennedy's other qualifications are 21 hours of evaluation experience, continuing education units in domestic violence training, and six supervised evaluations. To remain on the panel, he must be reevaluated on these requirements every 2 years.

Although Dr. Kennedy is licensed in California and follows California's requirements for child custody evaluators, his expertise and method of conducting his evaluations, though not used by all evaluators, should be. Child custody evaluators have 90 days to conduct their assessments. At the end of those 90 days or sooner, Dr. Kennedy completes a 30-page report for the attorneys or the court. He might have been hired by the parties, their attorneys, or the court, but all sides will have stipulated to his expertise and agreed to his services. Overall, the goal is an objective assessment that is, according to the law, "in the best interest of the child" (California Family Code § 3011). Sometimes, the court or the attorneys attempt to manipulate the results, but maintaining objectivity while evaluating the parties, engaging the child, and utilizing various assessment instruments if warranted is of paramount importance. Within the general evaluation process, Dr. Kennedy also notes the importance of a cultural assessment. His manner is soft-spoken,

(continued)

(*continued*)

relaxed, and empathic. While this appears to be his standard demeanor, he makes the point that it is the best approach to conducting custody evaluations, as it has proved to be the best approach in talking to the parents and child or children.

Unfortunately, Dr. Kennedy recently resigned from the Family Law panel. Although child custody evaluators do not make decisions about which parent, if either, should have custody but only issue recommendations, Dr. Kennedy was threatened by an unhappy father after the court rendered its decision in a contentious case. It is the county's loss, but Dr. Kennedy continues to give back and currently trains forensic psychology students for their future careers.

IN THE NEWS

The usual child custody arrangement between similarly situated divorced parents will either give physical custody to one with visitation to the other or split the child's time between the parents' homes. On July 6, 2017, during a custody exchange, a man allegedly shot his ex-wife and her boyfriend who was at the scene. The mother of the couple's 9-year-old and 7-year-old was dead, and her boyfriend was badly wounded (Serna, 2017). Although custody issues are among the most emotional in family court, this couple had been divorced for several years, and no one questioned in the case seemed to know anything about problems. Most unfortunately, this is not an isolated story.

A very different kind of custody issue appeared on the same page of the local newspaper that same day. A mother left her four children locked in a hot car with the windows rolled up. When she realized law enforcement was nearing, she tried to drive the car away. She was unsuccessful and was taken into custody, and custody of the children was given to a family member (Rocha, 2017).

While the truth behind these stories will never be known, what is known is that there are many forensic psychologists with the experience and expertise to evaluate these situations. Unfortunately, unless there is a problem or an argument that comes to the attention of the authorities, the professionals are rarely called in to evaluate. The process is expensive and time consuming. Nevertheless, having evolved to recognizing same-sex marriage, three-parent families, and men being able to give birth, one would hope that society and the law will evolve even further to prevent potential problems and employ the appropriate professionals before the crisis occurs.

SUMMARY

This chapter provided an overview of forensic psychology in family court. The changing modern family and child custody issues were highlighted. Two areas that might be considered only collateral to family issues are domestic violence and suicide. Suicide was included in this chapter for several reasons: There is an upsurge of teen suicides, which includes children still living with their family of origin; suicide is a major research area for forensic psychologists; and forensic psychologists are in a particularly good position to conduct psychological autopsies when the circumstances require them. Domestic violence was included because even though it is not necessarily limited to family members, it is a problem that does occur in families; forensic psychologists may be called in to evaluate domestic violence either as a collateral issue to child custody issues or for direct evaluation and testimony. Dr. Clive Kennedy's interview not only explained the role of a family panel evaluator, but also confirmed the need for training in so many of the areas that family matters cover, both legally and psychologically.

DISCUSSION QUESTIONS

1. As a child custody evaluator, what questions would you want to ask the parties? What might you be looking for in individual and family interactions that might help you with your recommendations?
2. How might a psychological autopsy be standardized? Where would you start?

3. Although family matters have many topics and areas requiring the expertise of a forensic psychologist, are there enough commonalities to make some broad generalizations? What might they be?

4. *Painter v. Bannister* (1966) continues to have significance in family law for several reasons. Read the whole case. What do you think of the Iowa Supreme Court's decision and the reasoning behind it? Find the case at https://www.courtlistener.com/opinion/1281464/painter-v-bannister/.

NOTES

1. According to the majority opinion of the California Supreme Court in the *In Re Marriage Cases* (2008), what was then California Civil Code § 55 defined the age of consent as 18 for men and 15 for women. The code also defined marriage as a lifetime commitment.

2. In 1934, the Restatement of the Conflict of Laws (which seems to no longer be available) stated that a marriage valid where celebrated would be valid everywhere unless it violates the strong public policy of the forum state. The Restatement of Conflict of Laws 2nd added that the public policy being referred to was that of the state that had the most significant relationship with the marriage (Swisher et al., 2012).

3. California actually had a miscegenation law, which it had repealed in 1948 (*In re Marriage Cases*, 2008).

4. Although domestic partnerships had been recognized in California for almost two decades, in 1999 (Family Code §§ 497–499), the state enacted a formal domestic partnership law that gave same-sex couples similar state rights as married people. In 2005, more state rights and obligations were added to the act, but the explanation made very clear that a domestic partnership was not a marriage that would be recognized outside the state of California (Davidson, 2004).

5. By the time this case was decided, 37 states and the District of Columbia had legalized same-sex marriage.

6. As of this writing, five states (California, Colorado, Oregon, Vermont, Washington) and the District of Columbia have enacted death with dignity or assisted suicide statutes. All these laws require consultation with at least one mental health expert and the existence of a terminal

illness prior to allowing the lethal prescription. Although mental health experts have a role in those suicides, they are not part of this topic.

7. While the empirical evidence remains conflicting regarding motivation for suicide, the effect on family members is real. The instances cited in this chapter are not hypothetical and have been described by surviving relatives socially and professionally.

REFERENCES

Altafulla v. Ervin 238 Cal. App. 4th 571 (2015).

American Academy of Matrimonial Lawyers (2011). *Child custody evaluation standards*. Retrieved from http://www.aaml.org/sites/default/files/Standards_Child_Custody.pdf

Associated Press. (2017, June 19). Modern family: More courts allowing three parents of one child. *NBC News*. Retrieved from http://www.nbcnews.com/feature/nbc-out/modern-family-more-courts-allowing-three-parents-one-child-n774031

Bird, B. (n.d.). Which states are no fault divorce states? *Legalzoom*. Retrieved from http://info.legalzoom.com/states-nofault-divorce-states-20400.html

Brake, E. (2016). Marriage and domestic partnership. In E. N. Zalta (Ed.), *The Stanford encyclopedia of philosophy*. Retrieved from https://plato.stanford.edu/cgi-bin/encyclopedia/archinfo.cgi?entry=marriage

Brief for American Psychological Association, California Psychological Association, American Psychiatric Association, National Association of Social Workers, and National Association of Social Workers, California Chapter in Support of the Parties challenging the Exclusion. *In re Marriage Cases* S147999 (2008).

Buirski, N. (Producer), & Nichols, J. (Director). (2016). *Loving* [Motion picture]. United States: Raindog Films & Big Beach Films.

Bullying Statistics & Information. (2017). American Society for the Positive Care of Children. Retrieved from http://americanspcc.org/bullying/statistics-and-information/?gclid=CjwKCAjw2ZXMBRB2EiwA2HVD-A_kLJdN6hcU4ef2Z3_pp7qKyB05eZh6L_Fi6rOKpHa1RNaAKa3cfhoCgJoQAvD_BwE.

California Family Code § 2310-2313, 2335. (1970).

California Penal Code § 262.

California Probate Code §§ 810-12, 6100, 6100.5.

Canter, D. V. (2000). Psychological autopsies. *Encyclopaedia of Forensic Sciences*. Retrieved from http://eprints.hud.ac.uk/id/eprint/8669/

Cavanaugh, J. T., Carson, A. J., Sharpe, M., & Lawrie, S. M. (2003). Psychological autopsy studies of suicide: A systematic review. *Psychological Medicine*, *33*(3), 395–405.

Consent to Adoption by State (n.d.). Retrieved from http://www.abcadoptions.com/consent4.htm

Davidson, J. W. (2004). *AB 205 (The Domestic Partners Rights and Responsibilities Act of 2003) and its impact on cities.* League of California Cities. Retrieved from https://www.cacities.org/uploadedfiles/leagueinternet/93/93496734-f1e8-42a5-a267-90db956201e4.pdf

Edelman, A., & Katz, C. (2015, July 29). Trump lawyer Michael Cohen apologizes for reporter threats. *New York Daily News.* Retrieved from http://www.nydailynews.com/news/politics/ivana-trump-rejects-rape-allegations-article-1.2306290

Fielder, M. (Producer). (n.d.). *The six wives of Henry VIII* [Video series]. New York, NY: Granada Bristol Productions. Retrieved from http://www.pbs.org/wnet/sixwives/about/schedule.html

Foster, T. (2011). Adverse life events proximal to adult suicide: A synthesis of findings from psychological autopsy studies. *Archives of Suicide Research, 15*(1), 1–15.

Frank, G. J. (2017). *Step-parent and non-parent rights.* Retrieved from http://www.garyfranklaw.com/Practice-Areas/Step-Parent-and-Non-Parent-Rights.shtml

Goodridge v. Mass. Department of Public Health. 440 Mass. 309 (2003).

Grace, R. M. (2010, June 24). Divorce law in early days: A whole lot different. *Metropolitan News-Enterprise,* 15.

Griswold v. Connecticut (1965).

Grossman, J. L. (2015, April 28). Interstate marriage recognition: When history meets the Supreme Court. *Verdict.* Retrieved from https://scholarlycommons.law.hofstra.edu/faculty_scholarship/644

Gutheil, T. G. (2007). Common pitfalls in the evaluation of testamentary capacity. *Journal of the American Academy of Psychiatry and the Law, 35*(4), 514–517.

Harper, J. (2013, September 17). Bullying, mobbing and the role of shame. *Psychology Today.* Retrieved from https://www.psychologytoday.com/blog/beyond-bullying/201309/bullying-mobbing-and-the-role-shame

In re Marriage Cases No. S147999 (May 15, 2008).

In re Matter of Baby M. 109 N.J. 396 (1988).

Lawrence, R. E., Oquendo, M. A., & Stanley, B. (2015). Religion and suicide risk: A systematic review. *Archives of Suicide Research, 20*(1), 1–21.

Lee, L., Roser, M., & Ortiz-Ospina, E. (2016). *Suicide.* OurWorldInData.org. Retrieved from https://ourworldindata.org/suicide/

Lloyd, J. (2013, June 28). Supreme Court clears way for same-sex marriage in California [Video]. *NBC News.* Retrieved from http://www.nbclosangeles.com/news/local/California-Same-Sex-Marriage-Prop-8-Supreme-Court-211812241.html

Loving v. Virginia 388 U.S. 1 (1967).

Luxton, D. O., June, J. D., & Fairall, J. M. (2012). Social media and suicide: A public health perspective. *American Journal of Public Health, 102*(2), 195–200.

Malesky, B. (2012, June 21). Divorce: Dilemma for early Americans. *Archives.* Retrieved from http://www.archives.com/experts/malesky-betty/divorce-in-family-history-research.html

Moskos, M., Olson, L., Halbern, S., Keller, T., & Gray, D. (2005). Utah youth suicide study: Psychological autopsy. *Suicide & Life-Threatening Behavior, 35*(5), 536–546.

New York Domestic Relations Law (DRL). §§ 170-170.7.

Obergefell v. Hodges 135 S.Ct.2071 (2015).

Painter v. Bannister 140 N.W. 2d 152 (1966).

Pappas, S. (2015, June 23). Social media cyber bullying linked to teen depression. *Scientific American.* Retrieved from https://www.scientificamerican.com/article/social-media-cyber-bullying-linked-to-teen-depression/

Parenting in America. (2015, December 17). Pew Research Center. Retrieved from http://www.pewsocialtrends.org/2015/12/17/parenting-in-america/

Perlin, M. L., Champine, P., Dlugacz, H. A., & Connell, M. (2008). *Competence in the law: From legal theory to clinical application.* Hoboken, NJ: Wiley & Sons.

Rocha, V. (2017, July 7). Mother is arrested after 4 children are locked in a hot car. *Los Angeles Times,* B4.

Rouleau, W. C. (October 22, 2016). The truth about suicide & life insurance. *Huffington Post.* Retrieved from http://americanspcc.org/bullying/statistics-and-information/?gclid=CjwKCAjw2ZXMBRB2EiwA2HVD-A_kLJdN6hcU4ef2Z3_pp7qKyB05eZh6L_Fi6rOKpHa1RNaAKa3cfho CgJoQAvD_BwE

Rushing, E. (2016). Recent changes in testamentary capacity rules. *JAMS.* Retrieved from https://www.jamsadr.com/files/uploads/documents/articles/rushing-thebarjournal-recent-changes-in-testamentary-capacity-rules-spring-2016.pdf

Sachs, C., & Gomberg, L. (2004). Health effects of domestic violence. *Women's Rx. Newsletter of the Iris Cantor–UCLA Women's Health Education and Resource Center,* Los Angeles, CA.

Sachs, C., & Gomberg, L. (2009). Intimate partner sexual abuse. In C. Mitchell & D. Anglin (Eds.), *Intimate partner violence: A bio-psycho-social approach.* New York, NY: Oxford University.

Serna, J. (2017, July 7). Charges foiled against man in ex-wife's killing. *Los Angeles Times,* B4.

Smernoff, B. F. (1996). California's conclusive presumption of paternity and the expansion of unwed fathers' rights. *Golden Gate University Law Review, 26*(2), 237–368.

Snider, J. E., Hane, S., & Berman, A. L. (2006). Standardizing the psychological autopsy: Addressing the *Daubert* standard. *Suicide & Life Threatening Behavior, 36*(5), 511–518.

Stout, D. (2004, February 12). San Francisco city officials perform gay marriages. *New York Times*. Retrieved from http://www.nytimes.com/2004/02/12/national/san-francisco-city-officials-perform-gay-marriages.html

Swisher, P. N., Miller, A., & Shapo, H. S. (2013). *Family law: Cases, materials, and problems* (3rd ed.). [Kindle version]. LexisNexis. Retrieved from https://www.amazon.com/Family-Law-Cases-Materials-Problems-ebook/dp/B009I3JXUS/ref=mt_kindle?_encoding=UTF8&me=

Taylor, S. (2012). Testamentary capacity and undue influence in will contests. *LexisNexis Legal Newsroom*. Retrieved from https://www.lexisnexis.com/legalnewsroom/estate-elder/b/estate-elder-blog/archive/2012/02/01/testamentary-capacity-and-undue-influence-in-will-contests.aspx?Redirected=true

Teen suicide. (2013, October). American Academy of Child & Adolescent Psychiatry. Retrieved from https://www.aacap.org/aacap/families_and_youth/facts_for_families/fff-guide/Teen-Suicide-010.aspx

United States v. Windsor 570 U.S. ___(2013).

Weisbrod, C. (2006). *Painter v. Bannister*: Still. *Utah Law Review*. Faculty Article and Papers 100. Retrieved from http://digitalcommons.uconn.edu/cgi/viewcontent.cgi?article=1099&context=law_papers

Zadrozny, B., & Mak, T. (2015, July 27). Ex-wife: Donald Trump made me feel "violated" during sex. *Daily Beast*. Retrieved from http://www.thedailybeast.com/ex-wife-donald-trump-made-me-feel-violated-during-sex

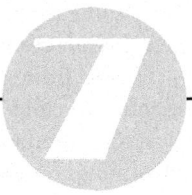

The Forensic Psychologist's Role in the Juvenile Justice System

OVERVIEW

The only theme of this chapter is a continuation of one of the themes in Chapter 6. Whenever the welfare of children is at issue, the state, federal government, and all interested individuals are charged with acting in **the best interest of the child** (see, for example, California Family Code § 3011, 1992; Illinois Compiled Statutes 750, 2016). As discussed in Chapter 6, this includes not only custody but also the more basic **child abuse, neglect,** and **abandonment.** The laws also take into account the behavior of the child. While specific age demarcations, acts, and punishments may vary, all states have separate **juvenile justice systems** that have certain commonalities requiring the input of forensic psychologists. Forensic psychologists may be called upon to evaluate pre- and/or post-disposition offending juveniles as well as to counsel those on **parole** or **probation**. By evaluating these minors, the forensic psychologist is in the best professional position to recommend education, rehabilitation, and treatment.

Aside from guidance in the case of a neglected, abused, or abandoned child or an offending juvenile, the forensic psychologist plays an important role in advocating for special needs children and advocating, on their behalf, enforcement of the antidiscrimination laws that apply to the educational system. Several cases illustrate the particular application of varying laws to various juvenile situations: *Larry P. v. Riles* (1979) is discussed, and *Roper v. Simmons* (2005) and *Miller v. Alabama* (2012) are revisited to introduce two other cases.

Some of the work of Thomas Grisso, PhD, and Laurence Steinberg, PhD, both prolific researchers and authors in matters related to the juvenile mind, will also be referenced, along with others whose work has advanced the forensic psychology of juveniles.

HOW IT WORKS

Juvenile law has a long and inconsistent history in the United States. Even the definition and subtopics vary according to whom is doing the defining. Further, except for the theorists who are famous for having studied their development, individuals under the age of majority are often interchangeably referred to as children, adolescents, juveniles, or minors.[1] The law distinguishes certain age ranges but often refers to anyone under the age of majority as an infant (see, for example, New York Consolidated Laws § 140(b), 2017). Keeping that in mind, another fact to remember is that although parents are expected to take care of their children until they at least reach the age of majority, the state, too, has a role. The state acts as **parens patriae**, meaning parent of the country, when its citizens cannot take care of themselves. This is the theory on which most juvenile law is based: The court, acting for the state and in place of the parent, will take care of its dependents (Sankaran, 2009).

So, for the purpose of the all-inclusive discussion of this chapter, the parameters will be broad and rely on a dictionary definition of juvenile law. This chapter addresses "that area of the law that deals with the actions and well-being of persons who are not yet adults" (Juvenile Law, 2008, para. 1). In Chapter 6, the well-being of the child in regard to custody was discussed. Here, the child's well-being in regard to treatment and education will be the topic. Then, the child's actions or behavior will be examined in relation to the juvenile justice systems that exist in all jurisdictions, as well as what the United States (U.S.) Supreme Court has had to say on the topic.

Abuse, Neglect, and Abandonment

Deciding whether or where to address child abuse in this book took some careful thought. Maltreatment of children is not among the first topics considered when thinking about the work of a forensic psychologist. Children who suffer from maltreatment usually find their way into the care of social services departments, which may be called Child Protective Services (CPS) or Dependent Children and Family Services (DCFS) depending upon the state, and their care is usually entrusted to a case worker (see, for eample, California Welfare & Institutions Code § 300 et seq., 1937). At least one state, California, requires its judges to have specialized training (2018 California Rules of Court). Further, while state codes make reference to social workers as case managers, the social workers are required to call in clinical experts, such as psychologists, to help determine appropriate placement and treatment for the dependent child (California Welfare & Institutions Code § 370, 1937). All of these cases end up in a juvenile court, and the forensic psychologist is the mental health expert who is familiar with court processes and able to guide this process (American Psychological Association, 2013).

Since 1974, a federal law has been in place to fund state research and community projects encouraging local involvement in preventing and remedying child maltreatment. The Child Abuse Prevention and Treatment Act was the result of a grass-roots effort of caring individuals, communities, and private agencies in response to a need for federal oversight of child maltreatment (National Child Abuse and Neglect Training and Publications Project, 2014). Its goal was prevention, but little was known about the incidence in individual states.

By 1967, all states had some form of mandatory reporting of child abuse and neglect, but the reporting was inconsistent both in requirements and in practice, making it difficult to understand or even compile the information needed to help resolve the problem. The goal was prevention, but the first and ongoing steps included funding evidence-based research—specifically, grants that would train professionals in the law, medicine, and others to engage in projects that would be focused on preventing and treating child abuse and neglect. This funding would be accomplished through the states participating in a national study to gather statistics on child abuse and neglect. An advisory board was formed to assure coordination and consistency (National Child Abuse and Neglect Training and Publications Project, 2014).

The Child Abuse Prevention and Treatment Act and its projects have been reauthorized for over 40 years by several presidential administrations, with added causes including all forms of domestic violence (Sedlak et al., 2010). Currently, the projects resulting from the Act and its successors are administered through the Department of Health and Human Services (DHHS). What makes this relevant for forensic psychology is that the goals have not changed. States are funded to engage in evidence-based research, to develop treatment and prevention projects, and to participate at the national level in coordinating, reporting, and punishing those persons who engage in child abuse of any kind.

In California, for example, the Child Abuse and Neglect Reporting Act (CANRA) (1980) is contained in the Penal Code. It not only lists all acts that are child abuse, but also lists mandatory reporters and includes a controversial section that became law in 2014 (Penal Code § 1165.1(c)(1)). Should a client reveal to a therapist that he or she views child pornography, that therapist is mandated to report it to law enforcement. Mental health professionals in the state sued to have the statute repealed as having a chilling effect on therapy. The California Supreme Court disagreed and said a person committing an illegal act should have no expectations of confidentiality and privacy and that watching child pornography is contributing to child sexual abuse (*Mathews v. Harris*, 2017).

The last major project was the Fourth National Incidence Study of Child Abuse and Neglect (NIS-4) in 2010 (National Child Abuse and Neglect Training and Publications Project, 2014). It was a collaboration of psychologists, researchers, statisticians, social workers, probation officers, teachers, and others investigating and compiling information on the incidence of individual child abuse throughout the country (Sedlak et al., 2010). They used standardized measures to compile and interpret their data, and the data included emotional abuse, physical abuse, and sexual abuse. Forensic psychologists are uniquely trained for participation in this type of study, and the published results leave no doubt as to the relevance of the work. The report is also clear that skilled professionals are needed to research and create programs for and with national organizations and agencies or through the states that are funded and do the reporting.[2]

Education

Although by not mentioning it, the Constitution originally left the education of the minor citizens up to the individual states, in 1975 Congress had passed the first Education for All Handicapped Children Act (EHA), and the federal courts were "forced … to enter that complicated area" (in *Larry P. v. Riles*, 1979, para. 3). The history of public education in the United States deserves and has been addressed in many volumes entirely devoted to the topic. However, for their relevance to forensic psychology, one federal law and its amendments and one case will tell the story.

EHA 1975 → IDEA 2004

A brief history of the EHA (1975) and its amendments over the next 30 or so years until it became the Individuals with Disabilities Education Act (IDEA, 2004) gives the context for the psycholegal issues with which mental health professionals, medical doctors, educators, parents, and the law are involved in the education of children. The overarching problem was that too many children were being denied an appropriate public education due to what were then called handicaps (EHA, 1975). EHA's stated purpose was to provide appropriate education for at least 1 million handicapped children who were not in school or were not receiving the special education they needed (EHA, 1975). The statute recognized that the states could not afford to create these special environments and to hire the more highly trained individuals required to effectively teach these children. Therefore, EHA provided that states that "established priorities for providing a free appropriate public education to all handicapped children" would receive federal funding for the project (§ 612 (3)).

By 2004, the EHA had been amended several times and became the IDEA. This last version of the act recognizes that the goals of the original act and amendments have not been achieved and goes so far as to provide legal penalties for states that do not comply with mandates for the free appropriate education. Children with disabilities are entitled to Individual Education Plans (IEP), being taught in the least restrictive environment, and having all reasonable accommodations made to provide their education; these interventions should begin at birth if disabilities are identified and continue through age 26 if necessary (IDEA, 2004). Further, the IEP is a team effort that includes the parents, educators, administrators, and school psychologists and other mental health professionals.

IDEA further recognized that some school districts were placing minority and immigrant students in special education classes in disproportionate numbers. Aside from raising the standards for special education teachers and accountability in general, IDEA provides that if it is determined that children are being placed in special education classes for reasons other than a disability, the state will be denied a percentage of its disability funding. This last was a direct reaction to findings that children whose English skills were poor due to immigrant status and other culturally limited but not educationally disabled students had been placed in special education classes (IDEA, 2004). Although the schools have been restricted from this arbitrary placement of students in special education classes, the practice continues. The decision in *Larry P. v. Riles* (1979) should have put a stop to this type of placement.

Larry P. v. Riles (1979)

Facts: The California schools had a disproportionate number of black students in special education classes in elementary schools. Specifically, black children were 10% of the total California school population but were 25% of the population of educatable mentally retarded (EMR) classes. Larry P. was one of those students, as were the other plaintiffs who made up the class that was suing the State of California through the Superintendent of Public Instruction and others for violating their constitutional rights of equal protection and due process. The weight of the evidence showed that the placement in these classes was based primarily on their scores on one intelligence test, the Stanford-Binet Intelligence Scale. The record did not show that the test had been normed on minority or immigrant populations.

The opinion provided a detailed history of intelligence testing, research based on intelligence testing, and California's application of the testing in the schools. The history revealed that no tests used up until that time had been normed on minority populations. Dr. David Wechsler, who developed intelligence tests for children and adults, had stated 35 years earlier that his tests could not be validly used for nonwhite populations, as his tests at the time were standardized on white populations.[3]

Some Special Terminology: This case was a **class action** requesting **certification** and **declaratory** and **injunctive relief**. First, classes must be certified by the court to continue as such. Briefly, this is accomplished by showing the court there is an identifiable group whose members are limited, similarly situated, and capable of being notified of the action. The federal district court for the Northern District of California certified the class as "all black San Francisco school children who have been classified as mentally retarded on the bases of IQ test results" (*Larry P. v. Riles*, 1979, II. Procedural Background, para. 1). Declaratory relief merely asks that the court make a statement as to the status of the parties. Here, the court certified the class. An injunction is basically a stop order. The plaintiffs were asking the court to make the school district stop placing the children in special education classes based on IQ tests.

Procedural History: The procedural history of the case reveals more about the background and issues. The original case was filed in federal district court in 1971 by a group of black students and their families from San Francisco. They stated the local and state defendants had violated their constitutional equal protection rights by incorrectly placing the children in EMR classes based on an IQ test score. The court granted a preliminary injunction, necessitating a complete investigation to determine whether the stop would be permanent; the order was issued in 1972.

In 1974, after the defendants appealed the preliminary injunction order, and it was affirmed for plaintiffs, the plaintiffs were allowed to expand their class to include all similarly situated California school children. The injunction was also expanded to include all black children and to prevent any school district from administering any test for placement that did not include accountability for cultural differences. In 1975, the state voluntarily stopped IQ testing for placement in EMR classes for all children. Rather than that resolving the issues, new state and federal legislation led the plaintiffs to amend their complaint, citing violations not only of the United States (U.S.) Constitution, but of the California Constitution and the California Education Code. In 1977, the U.S. Justice Department was allowed to participate as amicus curiae, "a friend of the court," to assert the position that IQ testing violates the EHA (1975); the plaintiffs again amended their complaint to reflect that same position (*Larry P. v. Riles*, 1979). Once back in federal district court, all motions by defendants to dismiss and for summary judgment were denied, and there was a trial on the merits. This is the federal district court opinion after the trial.

Issue: Is there any educational justification for the disproportionate number of black children in EMR classes in elementary schools in California?

Holding: Using any one test as the primary basis for determining a child is mentally retarded[4] violates equal protection of the U.S. and California Constitutions, the EHA (1975), parts of the Civil Rights Act of 1964, and California's Education Code. No test that does not take cultural diversity into consideration should be administered in public schools. This, in effect, is racial discrimination.

Judgment: For plaintiffs, with the injunction against using IQ tests for placement continuing in place.

A True Story

Many years ago, prior to the proliferation of computers and social media, a fifth grade class was reading a story about a middle-class family's daily experiences. The elementary school was located in a mostly minority, low socioeconomic status (SES) community. After they finished reading the story, a child raised his hand and asked the teacher if there was really such a thing as a car with a swimming pool in it, and how big would that car have to be. The teacher was momentarily stymied until she realized that the mother in the story had driven a "car pool." Not only did her students learn a new term that day, but the teacher learned a life lesson: Most of the families of the students in her class did not even own a car.

Juvenile Justice

Although custody, abuse, neglect, abandonment, and education are all topics for juvenile law in one way or another, they are all areas not driven by actions of the children. That is, they are driven by the actions of the adults and their effect on the children. Juvenile justice, however, is a topic that deals with juveniles who from their own actions become part of the juvenile justice system. The system is neither civil nor criminal, and every state has its own form. The juvenile justice systems were traditionally considered more civil than criminal, a possible reason juvenile offenders were historically denied constitutional rights (Bartol & Bartol, 2015; *In re Gault*, 1967). However, there are now federal mandates about treatment of juveniles that have evolved from false presumptions that children have no constitutional rights to carefully delineating the importance of assuring children are afforded their constitutional rights (*In re Gault*, 1967).

In 1967, the U.S. Supreme Court, in an 8–1 vote, decided that accused juvenile offenders were entitled to the same rights of due process, notice, services of an attorney, appeal, and warnings against self-incrimination as were adults. Gerald Gault was 15 years old and on probation when he was arrested for making an obscene phone call in Arizona. Because the Arizona juvenile justice system operated under the theory that proceedings involving children were more civil than criminal and that children had no rights except those of the state's parens patriae custody and protection, Gault's parents were not notified, he was held in detention for 2 months without a hearing, and he was not given the services of an attorney. Eventually, he was given 6 years in a juvenile facility for an act that an adult would have been punished with either a small fine or at most 2 months in jail (*In re Gault*, 1967).

Gault's case changed juvenile justice in the United States. Although juvenile offenses and juvenile dispositions are different in many cases from those of adults, because of *In re Gault* (1967) juvenile offenders are entitled to notice, hearings, a presumption of innocence, a right against self-incrimination, the right to confront an accuser, the right to an attorney, and all due process rights of adults. As will be seen, however, having the same rights as adults does not necessarily mean juveniles should receive the same punishment as adults. The law is continually trying to keep up with psychology to understand and account for differences in adolescent behavior and the adolescent mind (Steinberg, 2014).

Although *In re Gault* (1967) provides generally for the methods and processes all states must utilize in their juvenile justice systems, states vary within those parameters in terminology, age distinctions, and dispositions for certain acts. Further, states change their juvenile justice programs to comply with state and federal mandates as well as evolving science. California's juvenile justice system, for example, was the California Youth Authority until the early 2000s. At that time, it was recognized the name had a negative connotation, and if the juvenile justice system was going to be reformed, it needed its name changed as well (Farrell Litigation Timeline, 2013). Illinois, the first state to introduce a juvenile court in 1899, revised the goals of its juvenile justice system almost 100 years later in 1998, with the Illinois Juvenile Court Act (Bostwick, 2010). The largest change was that the principles of restorative justice became the "guiding philosophy for the Illinois juvenile justice system," with the three main goals being accountability, community safety, and competency development (Bostwick, 2010, p. 1; Choi, Bazemore, & Gilbert, 2012).[5]

Terminology and philosophy aside, most juvenile justice systems are similar in practice, although the divisions, dispositions, or age distinctions may differ. California's system is not unusual and is comprehensive in its scope. It has been both lauded and vilified at various times and serves as a representative framework to explain the systems (Farrell Litigation Timeline, 2013). Most of the laws pertaining to the topic of juveniles in California are contained in the state's Welfare and Institutions Code. When the behavior of the youth is such that the law needs to step in and take custody of the juvenile, rather than being called a dependent (§§ 300 et seq.), the youth becomes a ward (§§ 601–608).

Juvenile Delinquency

While children have been determined to have the constitutional protections that adults enjoy, children continue to require the state to act as parens patriae in various situations. Certain privileges and obligations do not attach to children. For example, individuals under the age of 18 cannot vote and are not subject to selective service registration (Steinberg, 2014). The states also regulate the age at which individuals can legally marry, drink, drive, and smoke cigarettes. These laws are all enacted in the best interest of the child. Sometimes, as in the case of drinking, the laws are extended to an age over that of majority in the best interest of the child.

In addition, laws are enacted creating status crimes, which are so designated because they have been committed by a minor. In California, these acts include school truancy and breaking a curfew. Specifically, the law states the child can be adjudged a ward if it is determined that the child consistently "refuses to obey" reasonable orders of parents or guardians. These children come under the jurisdiction of the juvenile court according to § 601 of the Welfare and Institutions Code and may be referred to special programs established by other sections of the Code. Although the court may keep jurisdiction, the Code cautions that whenever possible these children should be left in the care of their parents or guardians. However, if the minor becomes a chronic "601" offender, the court may consider him or her as a "602" offender.

Juvenile Crimes

Section 602 offenders are described as children whose acts, if they were adults, would be crimes. Juvenile offenders who commit heinous crimes have presented almost unresolvable problems for the U.S. justice system. The states and the courts have vacillated in their policies between rehabilitation and punishment as the ultimate goal of juvenile justice in an effort to reduce juvenile crime (Hinton, Sims, Adams, & West, 2007). Although housing juveniles with adult offenders was recognized as detrimental to the juvenile at the beginning of the 19th century, until Illinois developed the first juvenile justice court at the end of that century, juvenile offenders were treated as adults within the criminal justice system (Bostwick, 2010).

Tried in Criminal Court

Throughout the 20th century, researchers, the public, and the courts sought the most effective ways to reduce juvenile crime rates (Grisso et al., 2003). In the process, the age at which juveniles could be tried in criminal courts was lowered and the acts for which they could be tried were expanded (Grisso et al., 2003). During this time, California amended its Welfare and Institutions Code § 602 to mandate that all juveniles age 14 and over be tried in criminal court if they were alleged to have committed any of a list of specific heinous crimes (see former § 602 (b); Gorman, 1995). Of course, being tried in criminal court did not mean the child would be housed with adults if found guilty; it did, however, mean that the child could and would be prosecuted and sentenced as an adult. During the years of minority, the child would be kept in a juvenile detention setting; once juvenile court jurisdiction ended, however, if the child's sentence was not complete, the rest of the sentence would be spent in jail or prison with adults. What was not considered was that psychological research showed that most 14-year olds were not competent to assist in their own trial, nor did they fully comprehend the nature of the proceedings (*Dusky v. United States*, 1960; Grisso et al., 2003).

In 2006, a comprehensive study of juvenile victims and offenders by the Department of Justice sought to gather enough statistics to be able to make some generalizations about juvenile offenders (Snyder & Sickmund, 2006). What the researchers found was that many juvenile offenses go unreported, states vary in age distinctions regarding juvenile court jurisdiction, and there are no reliable juvenile recidivism rates. Some states report recidivism, while some report success. Generally, those juveniles on probation recidivate with less frequency than those who are incarcerated. The authors logically attributed that difference to the fact that the probationers had likely committed lesser crimes to begin with than the inmates. Unfortunately, this seems to be the last compilation of these types of data, and the statistics regarding juveniles and their treatment in the law change frequently. The final statement made in the report on the state of juvenile justice was that the trend in the United States, at least in 2006, seemed to be to hold juvenile offenders less culpable than their adult counterparts (Snyder & Sickmund, 2006).

An example of the changing attitudes and policies regarding juvenile justice can be found in the same California statute that created the mandatory filing in adult court of certain 14-year-old offenders two decades earlier (Gorman, 1995; Public Safety and Rehabilitation Act, 2016). In 2016, when Proposition 57 went to the voters of California, they voted to eliminate mandatory filing of charges in criminal court for trial if the juveniles were 14 or over and accused of certain crimes. As of January 1, 2017, rather than mandating the prosecution to file, the decision belongs to the judge after the prosecution makes a motion and an investigation is completed (Public Safety and Rehabilitation Act, 2016). The judge has the discretion to take several enumerated factors into consideration in making this decision. However, if the juvenile is 14 or 15 years old, he or she can be tried as an adult only if the accusation is one of several listed crimes. In making the determination, the judge, among other things, "may give weight" to the juvenile's past behavior, mental state, services previously provided to the child, and mental and emotional development. It goes without saying that a mental health professional would be the only person qualified to conduct such an investigation for the court.

Disposition

When juveniles are found guilty of offenses in juvenile court, the next step is referred to as "disposition," rather than "sentencing." Disposition of a case depends upon the jurisdiction, crime, age of the juvenile, and delinquent history. Once tried in juvenile court, if the juvenile is sent to a facility, the term cannot be longer than the juvenile court's jurisdiction, however much longer that might be. This sometimes questionable practice was illustrated when Ethan Couch, then 16 years old, killed four people in 2013. Ethan was driving with a blood alcohol level over two times the legal limit while on an alcohol run to add to the supply at a party that was under way at his Texas home. According to the reports, Ethan was living alone in this very large house while his parents were living elsewhere.

During his trial in juvenile court, Ethan's psychologist testified that Ethan was suffering from "affluenza"—that he was rich and spoiled and knew no better. The judge, whether swayed by the testimony or for whatever reason, sentenced Ethan to inpatient treatment and 10 years' probation rather than incarcerating him. Ethan violated his probation, and the concern was that because Texas keeps jurisdiction only until a juvenile is 19, Ethan would not have to serve any jail or prison time. However, due to the probation violation, when Ethan turned 18 the juvenile court judge was able to transfer his case to the criminal court. where the judge sentenced him to 2 years in jail (Tsiaperas, 2017).

The results have been quite different, however, for juveniles transferred to criminal court. As was seen in Chapter 4, up until the early years of this century, the sentencing of juveniles could be and was as harsh as that of adults. Juveniles were sentenced to death and life without the possibility of parole in states that allowed those sentences (*Roper v. Simmons*, 2005).

Research

The cases and the changing laws in so many civil and criminal cases show the work of forensic psychologists and others as they have continued their research into these controversial children- and adolescent-related areas. If the trend is or was toward holding the juvenile offender less culpable than the adult, it was most likely the result of the evidence-based research being conducted by experts in the field (Snyder & Sickmund, 2006).

Thomas Grisso

As mentioned in Chapter 4, Thomas Grisso began studying juveniles and their legal comprehension in the 1970s. By 1980, he had studied hundreds of incarcerated youth and concluded that the younger the juvenile, the less he understood the *Miranda* warnings and did not waive his rights knowingly. Grisso (1980) also concluded that just because older teens *seemed* to know their rights as well as adults, the standard was not high enough to assure that the teens did actually understand their rights. Two and a half decades later, he determined in collaboration with others that the same caveat applied to juveniles and their competency to stand trial: The younger the juvenile, the less competent he or she is to understand the nature of the proceedings (Grisso, 1980; Grisso et al., 2003).

Laurence Steinberg

Laurence Steinberg has written extensively about teens and their behavior. Much of his research is about the teen mind and motivation (Steinberg & Monahan, 2007). One of his areas of research is the teen's propensity to submit to peer pressure and engage in risky behavior. Similar to the conclusion reached by Grisso, Steinberg found that the younger the adolescent, the more likely the chance the teen would succumb to peer pressure and engage in risk-taking behavior. After studying through self-report and valid behavioral measures 935 ten- to thirty-year-old individuals, Steinberg and colleagues found that adolescents between the ages of 10 and 15 are the most likely to engage in sensation-seeking behaviors and that impulsivity declines and remains stable thereafter (Steinberg et al., 2008).

Since much of Steinberg's research seems to have led him to the conclusion that the adolescent mind hits some sort of plateau with respect to impulsivity and vulnerability by age 15, it is not terribly surprising that in 2014 he advocated allowing 16-year-olds to vote. In advocating for this right, Steinberg (2014) noted that many countries have lowered their voting age to 16 or 17 and that U.S. age demarcations are arbitrary. According to him, there is no science that can point to an age at which an individual leaves adolescence and becomes an adult, and distinctions should be made based on decisions he calls "cold cognition" or "hot cognition" (p. A 12). Cold cognition activities are those requiring decisions that can take time to be made; hot cognition decisions are those that require instant decisions. For the former, 16-year-olds can gather evidence and advice; for the latter (e.g., driving, drinking, and criminal responsibility), immediate decisions may be required, and the consequences could be life changing. Since voting requires only "cold cognition," according to Steinberg (2014), 16-year-olds can take their time to make a decision, and they may make "bad choices, but statistically speaking, they won't make them any more often than adults" (p. A 12).

Others

Modern technology and scientific understanding have led forensic researchers in directions that could not have been contemplated until the end of the last century (Bowman, 2004). While Steinberg (2014) may have been referring to technology when he mentioned the "science of adolescent development," others in the field have found that brain development may continue through the early and mid-20s. The use of functional magnetic resonance imaging (fMRI) has allowed researchers to map the brain and determine development and growth at certain chronological ages (Davies, 2004). The fMRI results show that the frontal lobe, called the prefrontal cortex, is the last part of the brain to develop (Davies, 2004). The function of this area of the brain is executive decision making and judgment, and studies show that this aspect of the brain continues to develop into the 20s (Johnson, Blum, & Giedd, 2009; Kassin et al., 2010). In fact, technology was not necessary when psychologist Yurgelun-Todd Deborah of Harvard Medical School showed cards of facial expressions to adults and adolescents (Packard, 2007). She found that while adults were able to correctly read facial expressions such as fear, adolescents could not (Bowman, 2004; Packard, 2007).

SPOTLIGHT ON CASES

While *Roper v. Simmons* (2005) and *Miller v. Alabama* (2012) were landmark decisions regarding the sentencing of juvenile offenders, they are statutorily resolved, with age at the time of the crime being the only determinant. Therefore, they were presented in Chapter 4 as part of the discussion of due process, equal protection, sentencing of certain individuals, and the limitations on states' rights (United States Constitution, 1791). One would think that a clear mandate that no one under the age of 18 years when the crime was committed could be sentenced to death or life in prison without the possibility of parole would end controversial sentencing, at least in federal courts. However, because of those rulings, the door seems to have opened for defendants to ask the courts to rethink their sentences.

These are not landmark decisions, but they do illustrate the creative thinking of the legal and psychological communities.

State v. Skakel (2006)

Facts: Martha Moxley was a 15-year-old girl found bludgeoned to death on her family's property in 1975. She knew the Skakel family and had stopped at their house with a friend after 9:00 p.m., the night of her murder. When she did not arrive home at 11:00 p.m., her mother eventually called the police. A neighbor found her body the next day. It appeared as if her body had been dragged after her head had been hit repeatedly with a golf club, parts of which were found nearby. Martha's pants had been pulled down and semen was found on her body, as was a stab wound from the golf club. The autopsy report judged the time of death to be close to 9:30 p.m. the night before her body was found.

The Skakel family members were all questioned at the time. Michael Skakel, who was also 15, stated he was with his siblings and did not leave the house after they all arrived home that night. Other evidence showed the murder weapon had come from the Skakel home. In 1977, Skakel attempted suicide, telling his family's driver that he had done something terrible and should die. From 1978 until 1980, he attended a school for troubled teens in Maine. While there, he allegedly told several people stories about the night of the murder that included his being drunk, not remembering, getting confused as to whether he or his brother committed the murder, and finally admitting he did it. In 1991, however, he recanted, saying he masturbated while sitting in a tree watching his brother make advances toward Martha. In 1997, he told a reporter he and Martha had made plans to go trick-or-treating together on the next night, which was Halloween, but that he had left his house to go sit in the tree.

Procedural History: At some point around 2000, Skakel was arrested for the murder of Moxley. Because Skakel was 15 at the time of the murder, charges were originally filed in Connecticut's Juvenile Court. The juvenile court judge transferred the case to criminal court after finding there was reasonable cause to believe the defendant committed the crime and ordering an investigation as required by statute.

Rule: All determinations must be made from the laws in effect at the time the crime was committed.

Issues: Were the requirements of transferring from juvenile to adult court followed in the case? Can a statute of limitations be retro-actively applied? Did the state withhold exculpatory evidence depriving the defendant of a fair trial? Was the admission of testimony of a deceased person in violation of the hearsay rule, thereby denying the defendant the right to face his accuser? Generally, do the facts reveal the defendant did not get a fair trial according to the state or U.S. Constitution or that prosecutorial misconduct led to the murder conviction?

Holding: First, although the investigation was not as complete as it would have been had the defendant been a minor at trial, it fulfilled the due process requirements. There was no way the inves-tigation could have revealed a suitable juvenile placement for a 40-year-old defendant, and the case did not satisfy an out-of-state placement at any time. If mental illness was an issue, the burden was on the defendant to raise it. Second, although the statute of limitations at the time was 5 years for prosecution for felonies, it did not expressly state murder was one of them. Further, the statute excluding murder from the 5-year limitation was enacted within a year of the trial, making it interpretable as an amendment to the original statute and not specifically making it retroactive. Third, it is the responsibility of the defendant to prove the state hid excul-patory evidence. Notice of the evidence in question was provided by the state in various documents prior to the verdict. At no time did the defendant request the evidence. Other potentially exculpa-tory evidence was not requested until sometime after verdict, and the judge did not abuse his discretion in denying it be turned over to the defendant. Fourth, the transcript reveals that the defendant had the opportunity to face his accuser at the probable cause hearing. Skakel's attorney cross-examined him intensely, and the testimony that was admitted at trial was that testimony. No part of the record reflects prosecutorial misconduct. The prosecution is entitled to ask the jury to make logical assumptions.

Judgment: Affirmed for the state. Michael Skakel had been sentenced to 20 years to life for the murder of Martha Moxley.

Epilogue(s): In 2013, Skakel's murder conviction was overturned based on inadequate legal representation. Skakel's new attorneys contend that the first one had not properly requested exculpatory evidence, did not introduce alibi evidence, and never mentioned reasonable doubt (Cowan & Santora, 2013). The state appealed the overturning of the conviction. In 2016, the Connecticut Supreme Court reinstated it, stating that according to the record Skakel's attorney had performed on every point made (Feuer & Hussey, 2016). Although the reinstatement of his sentence was finalized in early 2017, as of May 2017, Skakel was not returned to prison (Associated Press [AP], 2017b).

Lee Boyd Malvo (The Beltway Sniper)

Facts: Court reports and records are unavailable for this case, as there was really no contest. In 2002, Lee Boyd Malvo was arrested with an accomplice for 10 murders in Virginia, Maryland, and Washington, D.C. His accomplice was an adult when the acts occurred, but Malvo was 17 years old. The accomplice, John Muhammed, was tried, convicted, sentenced to death, and executed in 2009. Malvo was tried in Virginia, and although the prosecution had asked for the death penalty, the jury returned a sentence of life without the possibility of parole. In Maryland, he waived his right to an appeal and accepted a sentence of life imprisonment (AP, 2017a).

Issue: Should the ruling in *Miller v. Alabama* (2012) and its retroactive application be applicable to an individual who pleaded guilty and negotiated a plea bargain for a sentence?

Holding: New sentencing hearings need to be held, as *Miller v. Alabama* (2012) grants rights to juveniles that did not exist when Malvo made his deal (AP, 2017). Therefore, John Malvo did not make a voluntary plea agreement.

Judgment: Almost 3 months after this report, there is no judgment regarding a new sentencing hearing in this case.

FOCUS ON CAREERS

Dr. Sammie Williams received his PsyD degree in forensic psychology and became a licensed clinician in 2007. During his training, he worked at Metropolitan State Hospital and Juvenile Justice Centers. Through Child Protective Services (CPS) he began evaluating children of all ages for developmental and mental health issues. These children were already in the system and not in parental custody. Moving on to the Department of Mental Health, Dr. Williams developed extensive experience and professional satisfaction; he remained employed in that organization for several years.

Eventually, Dr. Williams' professional life evolved into private practice specializing in diagnosis and treatment of at-risk children and their families. His referrals may come from CPS, schools, and physicians. Most recently, his practice has focused on identifying children with autism spectrum disorder (ASD), attention-deficit/hyperactivity disorder (ADHD), and other neurodevelopmental disorders. He has expertise in testing and evaluating, and many of his referrals come from psychiatrists. While these children are usually quite young, he is also called upon to identify cognitive challenges in adults.

Dr. Willliams has been called upon to testify as an expert on occasion, but he refuses to work for either "side" in a legal controversy. Although he turns down these requests, he remains available for neutral recommendations regarding juvenile fitness to be tried as an adult. In California, this is referred to as a "707 hearing" that must be conducted prior to transferring a juvenile to adult court (Public Safety and Rehabilitation Act, 2016; Welfare & Institutions Code). With the enactment of the Public Safety and Rehabilitation Act of 2016, and with transfer to adult court no longer mandated, requests for these evaluations will most likely become much more frequent.

IN THE NEWS

The general rule has always been that children remain in the custody of their parents as long as the parents have not abused, neglected, or abandoned them or unless the child's behavior is such that it is in the best interest of the child and society to remove the child from the parents' custody. On July 20, 2017, the California Supreme Court ruled that a child whose parent cannot control the behavior, through no fault of the parent, can be supervised by the juvenile court, and the parent can be denied custody (*In re J.T.,* 2017). Prior to this ruling, to become a dependent of the juvenile court, the parent had to have been found to be abusive, to be neglectful, or to have abandoned the child. In this instance, the mother stated her child was incorrigible, challenged the lower court's finding of dependency, and argued that her daughter belonged in a delinquency court rather than a dependency court (Egelko, 2017; *In re R.T.,* 2017). The premise here is that parents need to protect their children, and Welfare and Institutions Code § 300 implies this as part of the duty to not abuse, neglect, or abandon children (*In re R.T.,* 2017).

By the time this case was decided, R.T. was an adult and living with her grandparents. One can only assume that the mother's challenge to an earlier similar ruling had to do with her needing to make a statement that she was not at fault in her daughter's risky behavior. The court made clear that it made no judgment about the mother's behavior, but found only that the mother could not protect her child (*In re R.T.,* 2017).

SUMMARY

This chapter was all about children of all ages. With the exception of custody and parentage discussed in Chapter 6, all aspects of children and the law were discussed through laws, psychology, and cases. The approach was chronological, in that the first part of the chapter addressed abused, neglected, and abandoned children (usually the youngest), then considered education, and finished with the main forensic psychology topic of juveniles in the justice system—that is, delinquents; their behavior, rights, and punishment; and the laws that affect them. Research into the adolescent brain was cited, as were several topical cases that illustrate the still fluctuating thinking about juvenile justice. Finally, a profile of Dr. Sammie Williams, a forensic psychologist who specializes in diagnosing and treating at-risk juveniles, provided some insight into that forensic specialty.

DISCUSSION QUESTIONS

1. No one would dispute all children have a right to a "free and public education." However, IDEA (1990–2004), along with providing the education in the least restrictive environment, requires that the child with disabilities be educated in the same class as children without disabilities. This "mainstreaming" is a controversial topic. Discuss your thoughts about mainstreaming children with disabilities. Think about physical versus mental disabilities and psychological versus intellectual versus neurological disabilities.

2. The decision in *Larry P. v. Riles* (1979) not only set a standard for educational accountability and compliance, but also taught a strong lesson about diversity and cultural considerations. What are some issues about which today's schools/teachers need to be sensitive? Are they the same problems as in the latter part of the 20th century? Have those problems been resolved? Are they different?

3. Referring back to Chapter 4 and *Atkins v. Virginia* (2002) and *Hall v. Florida* (2014), and understanding that *Larry P. v. Riles* (1979) is about education, discuss specific reasons why these cases are reminiscent of each other.

NOTES

1. Erikson, Freud, and Piaget, to name just of few of the more well-known theorists, assigned probable age ranges to their theories of child development (King, Viney, & Woody, 2013).

2. This was a report made to Congress that is in the public domain. Credit, however, is given to the authors. The entire report can be found at: https://www.acf.hhs.gov/sites/default/files/opre/nis4_report_congress_full_pdf_jan2010.pdf.

3. The Wechsler intelligence tests continue to be updated and used for preschoolers (Wechsler Preschool and Primary Scale of Intelligence [WPPSI]), school children (Wechsler Intelligence Scales for Children [WISC]), and adults (Wechsler Adult Intelligence Scales [WAIS]). The current fifth version of the WISC was standardized on 2,200 age-appropriate children representative of the population based on gender, race/ethnicity, parent education level, and geographic location (Pearson Clinical). Retrieved from http://www.pearsonclinical.com/psychology/products/100000771/wechsler-intelligence-scale-for-childrensupsupfifth-edition--wisc-v.html/?utm_source=google&utm_medium=ppc&utm_campaign=3009632-D-701b00000006KgP&cmpid=701b00000006KgP#tab-details)

4. This was the court's term in 1975. It should also be noted that this was a district court decision. No party appealed the decision of the trial court.

5. Restorative justice is a construct used in forensic psychology as an area of research and practice. Its goal is to achieve resolution and healing by bringing the perpetrator and the victim or victim's survivors together for forgiveness and understanding of the perpetrator.

REFERENCES

American Psychological Association. (2013). Specialty guidelines for forensic psychology. *American Psychologist, 68*(1), 7–19. doi:10.1037/a0029889

Associated Press (AP). (2017a, May 8). Court issues final ruling reinstating Skakel conviction. Retrieved from https://www.usnews.com/news/best-states/connecticut/articles/2017-05-08/connecticut-court-to-release-ruling-on-kennedy-cousin-skakel

Associated Press (AP). (2017b, May 28). Judge overturns life terms of D.C. sniper. *Los Angeles Times*, A18.

Bartol, C. R., & Bartol, A. M. (2015). *Introduction to forensic psychology: research and application* (4th ed.). Thousand Oaks, CA: Sage.

Bostwick, L. (2010). *Policies and procedures of the Illinois juvenile justice system*. The Illinois Juvenile Justice Commission. Retrieved from http://www.icjia.state.il.us/assets/pdf/ResearchReports/IL_Juvenile_Justice_System_Walkthrough_0810.pdf

Bowman, L. (2004, May 11). New research shows stark difference in teen brains. *Scripps Howard News Service*. Retrieved from https://deathpenaltyinfo.org/new-research-shows-stark-differences-teen-brains

California Family Code § 3011 (1992).

California Welfare & Institutions Code, Division 2, §§ 200–742 (1937).

Child Abuse and Neglect Reporting Act (CANRA). Penal Code §§ 11464–11174.3 (1980).

Choi, J. J., Bazemore, G., & Gilbert, M. J. (2012). Review of research on victims' experiences in restorative justice: Implications for youth justice. *Children and Youth Services Review, 34*(1), 35–42.

Cowan, A. L., & Santora, M. (2013, November 21). After 11 years in prison, Skakel goes free on bail. *New York Times*. Retrieved from http://www.nytimes.com/2013/11/22/nyregion/skakel-is-ordered-free-on-bail.html?mtrref=undefined&gwh=D256467D0AD646953C0C71435828506C&gwt=pay

Davies, P. (2004, May 26). Psychiatrists question death for teen killers. *Wall Street Journal*. Retrieved from https://www.wsj.com/articles/SB108551562966820923

Dusky v. United States 362 U.S. 402 (1960).

Education of All Handicapped Children Act (EHA), 20 U.S.C. 1412 (1975).

Egelko, B. (2017, July 23). Kids who are out of control can be taken. *San Francisco Chronicle*, C1, C10.

Farrell Litigation Timeline. (2013). Center on Juvenile and Criminal Justice. Retrieved from http://www.cjcj.org/uploads/cjcj/documents/farrell_litigation_timeline_2015.pdf

Feuer, A., & Hussey, K. (2016, December 30). Michael Skakel's murder conviction has been reinstated. *New York Times*. Retrieved from https://www.nytimes.com/2016/12/30/nyregion/michael-skakels-murder-conviction-has-been-reinstated.html

Gorman, T. (1995, May 11). In law's eyes, 14-year-old is an adult: Crime: Under new state rule, boy could get life term if convicted of murder. *Los Angeles Times*. Retrieved from http://articles.latimes.com/1995-05-11/news/mn-65086_1_adult-court

Grisso, T. (1980). Juveniles' capacities to waive *Miranda rights*: An empirical analysis. *California Law Review, 68*(6), 1134–1166.

Grisso, T., Steinberg, L., Woolard, J., Cauffman, E., Scott. E., Graham S, … Schwartz, R. (2003). Juveniles' competence to stand trial: A comparison of adolescents' and adults' capacities as trial defendants. *Law and Human Behavior, 27*(4), 333–363.

Hinton, W. J., Sims, P. L., Adams, M. A., & West, C. (2007). Juvenile justice: A system divided. *Criminal Justice Policy Review, 18*(4), 466–483.

Illinois Compiled Statutes 750. Marriage and Dissolution of Marriage Act (2016).

In re Gault 387 U.S. I (1967).

In re R.T. S226416 (2017).

Individuals with Disabilities Education Act (IDEA), PL 20 U.S.C. 1400 (2004).

Johnson, S. B., Blum, R. W., & Giedd, J. N. (2009). Adolescent maturity and the brain: The promise and pitfalls of neuroscience research in adolescent health policy. *Journal of Adolescent Health, 45*(3), 216–221.

Juvenile law. (2008). *West's encyclopedia of American law* (2nd ed.). Retrieved from http://legal-dictionary.thefreedictionary.com/Juvenile+Law

Kassin, S. M., Drizin, S. A., Grisso, T., Gudjonsson, G. H., Leo, R. A., & Redlich, A. D. (2010). Police induced confessions: Risk factors and recommendations. *Law and Human Behavior, 34*(1), 3–38.

King, D. B., Viney, W., & Woody, W. D. (2013). *A history of psychology: Ideas and context* (5th ed.). New York, NY: Routledge.

Larry P. v. Riles 495 F. Supp.926 (N.D. Cal., 1979).

Mathews v. Harris 7 Cal. App. 5th 334 (2017).

Miller v. Alabama, 567 U.S. 460 (2012).

National Child Abuse and Neglect Training and Publications Project. (2014). *The Child Abuse Prevention and Treatment Act: 40 years of safeguarding America's children*. Washington, DC: U.S. Department of Health and Human Services, Children's Bureau.

New York Consolidated Laws. (2017). *Domestic Relations Law DOM § 140*. Retrieved from http://codes.findlaw.com/ny/domestic-relations-law/dom-sect-140.html

Packard, E. (2007). That teenage feeling. *Monitor on Psychology, 38*(4), 20. Retrieved from http://www.apa.org/monitor/apr07/teenage.aspx

Public Safety and Rehabilitation Act of 2016. Retrieved from https://www.gov.ca.gov/docs/The_Public_Safety_and_Rehabilitation_Act_of_2016_(00266261xAEB03).pdf

Roper v. Simmons, 543 U.S. 551 (2005).

Sankaran, V. (2009). Parens patriae run amuck: The child welfare system's disregard for the constitutional rights of non-offending parents. *Temple Law Review, 82*(1), 55–87.

Sedlak, A. J., Mettenburg, J., Basena, M., Petta, I., McPherson, K., Greene, A., & Li, S. (2010). *Fourth National Incidence Study of Child Abuse and Neglect (NIS-4): Report to Congress, executive summary*. Washington, DC: U.S. Department of Health and Human Services, Administration for Children and Families.

Snyder, H. N., & Sickmund, M. (2006). *Juvenile offenders and victims: 2006 national report*. Washington, DC: U.S. Department of Justice, Office of Justice Programs, Office of Juvenile Justice and Delinquency Prevention.

State v. Skakel. No 16844 (2006).

Steinberg, L. (2014, November 4). Science says let 16-year-olds vote. *Los Angeles Times*, A12.

Steinberg, L., Albert, D., Cauffman, E., Banich, M., Graham, S., & Woolard, J. (2008). Age differences in sensation seeking and impulsivity as indexed by behavior and self-report: Evidence for a dual systems model. *Journal of Developmental Psychology, 44*(6), 1764–1778.

Steinberg, L., & Monahan,.C. (2007). Age differences in resistance to peer influence. *Developmental Psychology, 43*(6), 1531–1543.

Tsiaperas, T. (2017, April 14). Ethan Couch will stay in jail after denial by state's highest court. *Dallas News.* Retrieved from https://www.dallasnews.com/news/crime/2017/03/20/affluenza-teens-attorneys-ask-texas-supreme-court-intervene-case

2018 California Rules of Court. (2018). *Standard 5.40 (e).* Retrieved from http://www.courts.ca.gov/cms/rules/index.cfm?title=standards&linkid=standard5_40

United States Constitution. (1789). Tenth Amendment (1791).

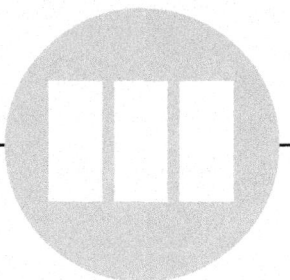

The forensic Psychologist and the Lawyer

While there is some thinking that conflict often exists between the roles of attorneys and forensic psychologists, the conflict—if it does exist—can be resolved by carefully distinguishing the differences in their roles, understanding the similarities in their disciplines, and emphasizing the need for mutual respect and dependence.

The Roles of the Forensic Psychologist and the Lawyer

OVERVIEW

This chapter distinguishes the roles of the attorney and the forensic psychologist by following their contributions from the pretrial stage through the course of a trial and to the post-trial proceedings. Also, it clarifies their roles and explains the ethical considerations of the forensic psychologist in regard to the question, "Who is the client?" The similarities and differences in the attorney's and the forensic psychologist's ethical codes, duties, and relationships are explored. Taking a cue from one of the attorneys interviewed for this chapter, an example of how each role is applied in the case of one legal construct is also explored. This construct is **"diminished capacity,"** which is no longer a defense in California and other states. The case that is recognized as the reason for the abolition of this defense, although over 30 years old, provides an excellent method for explaining the change.

The differences between the lawyer's **proof** and the psychologist's **probability** are addressed, as are the similarities in their ethical codes, investigative processes, and evidence presentation. To complete the understanding of the psychologist/attorney interaction and general relationship and to present it from a different perspective, interviews with two attorneys are provided. These attorneys—a criminal defense attorney and a family law certified specialist—represent the most frequent users of forensic psychologists for their cases.

For the sake of thoroughness, the potential roles of the clinical psychologist and the forensic psychologist in the courtroom setting are also distinguished. The presentation of another older, but landmark case illustrates that difference.

HOW IT WORKS

Although Chapter 4 presented the course of the trial, it did so from the perspective of a criminal trial and the potential for the employment of a forensic psychologist. Other chapters have referred to civil matters and how they progress through the legal system. What has not been done so far, however, is to address the actual application of the forensic psychologist's work through the perspective of the attorney. The attorney is the strategist of the case, and he or she makes the decisions regarding whom to bring in when. Some authors address the potential for conflict between the attorney and the psychologist, and many look to potential problems with the possible dual or conflicting roles of the psychologist during the course of the trial. However, their roles are delineated by their place in court, their ethical codes, and their experience.

The Example and a Case

While discussing the various and more obvious reasons a criminal defense attorney might call on a forensic psychologist, an old but specific example was mentioned—namely, "diminished capacity" (see the Stephan DeSales interview later in this chapter). Because looking at its application and the relevant case go beyond the scope of the interview discussion, and because expanding on the term "diminished capacity" is illustrative of how the forensic psychologist and the criminal defense attorney work as a team, an exploration of the case and the legal "fallout" from the case follow.

People v. White (1981)

Facts: George Moscone was mayor of San Francisco; Harvey Milk was a member of the Board of Supervisors, as was Dan White. White resigned his position, citing a work overload and inadequate compensation for supervisors. Within a few days, White changed his mind and notified the mayor, who led him to believe he would reappoint White. However, a newspaper reporter notified White that the mayor was going to appoint someone else the next day. On that day, White took a loaded gun, went to City Hall, sneaked in so he would not have to go through metal detectors, and walked in to the mayor's office, where he shot and killed Moscone. White then ran down the hallway to Milk's office, where they exchanged words and went to White's office. A few seconds later, witnesses said they heard gunshots. Both victims—Moscone and Milk—were shot multiple times, with some shots fired while the victims were incapacitated. At some point later that day, White surrendered to the police.

During his police interview White said he had been under a lot of pressure from home, politics, and finances, so he decided to resign his supervisor position. However, after informing his family of his resignation, he was told his family would support him in office. He then asked for reinstatement. He gave no reason for carrying a loaded gun, but said he got "fuzzy" with a "roaring" in his ears when the mayor confirmed he would not be reappointed, and he just shot him. Prior to going to Milk's office, White reloaded the gun and started thinking about how Milk was against him. When he saw Milk, he thought he was smirking at him, and he shot him.

At trial, the defense presented testimony from four psychiatrists and a psychologist. They all diagnosed White as being clinically depressed and generally without the present ability to premeditate. In other words, his capacity was diminished. One psychiatrist went so far as to say he could not form the intent to kill. The prosecution presented one psychiatrist who said White was moderately depressed.

Procedural History: Murder charges were filed against Dan White, and he had a jury trial. Unless expressly stated otherwise, lesser included offenses are automatically areas for a jury's consideration. **Voluntary manslaughter** is a lesser included offense in a trial for murder, in that it has the same result—that is, the death of a victim—and that the defendant did intend to kill. However, the elements of malice and premeditation were not proved beyond a reasonable doubt, as is the criminal burden. Dan White was convicted of voluntary manslaughter and sentenced for that crime. This case is the appeal of his sentence, which was at the upper limit of the term for voluntary manslaughter (7 years).

Special Terms: Murder is the premeditated, malicious, and intentional killing of one human being by another (California Penal Code § 187). A **lesser included offense** to murder would be voluntary manslaughter, a killing that was committed with intent but not with premeditation or malice (Calcagno, 1991; California Penal Code § 192).

Issue: Should mitigating factors be applied when the verdict is the lesser included charge so as to reduce the extensive length of the sentence?

Holding: The jury had enough facts to convict the defendant of first-degree murder, but did not. Therefore, the "diminished capacity" defense went to the verdict. The sentence is within the limits allowed by law for voluntary manslaughter.

Judgment: Affirmed.

The "Twinkie" Defense and Diminished Capacity

The case of Dan White caused a lasting controversy in California and beyond before, during, and after his trial and sentencing. He had shot and killed two elected city officials, having brought the loaded gun into the building with him. The controversy was created by the facts surrounding his defense of diminished capacity and the jury verdict, and resulted in a law being repealed. During the defense portion of the trial, his attorney questioned at least two witnesses, friends and colleagues of White, who testified among other things that when he was stressed, he seemed to abandon his usual lifestyle of healthy eating and exercise and to buy candy and other "junk food" on a regular basis (Linder, n.d.-a).

One of the psychiatric experts, whose credentials as a forensic psychiatrist were enumerated in the transcript, testified that White was regularly "gorging himself on junk food: Twinkies, Coca Cola" in response to direct examination (Linder, n.d.-b, 12th response). When questioned more specifically about the possibility of White's diminished capacity, Dr. Blinder stated that a high-sugar diet was probably one of three causes of White's diminished capacity. Without specifically citing any studies, Dr. Blinder further made a further statement about individuals whose criminal behavior stopped when they stopped eating junk food (Linder, n.d.-b).

Dan White's diminished capacity defense then became known as the "Twinkie defense" in the media (Krassner, 2011). Deservedly or not, it resulted in California abolishing the defense of diminished capacity to mitigate the crime (California Penal Code § 25[a], 1982). As was seen in White's trial, this was a defense that could be used successfully with the help of the forensic mental health professionals (Linder, n.d.-a). Unfortunately, even though several mental health professionals testified that he could not have premeditated the killings due to his depression, and a psychologist administered psychological tests and came to the same conclusion, what the public remembered about White's defense was that he ate junk food. In 1982, the voters of California overwhelmingly voted to abolish diminished capacity as a defense (California Penal Code §25 [a]; Weinstock, Leong, & Silva, 1996).

Epilogue: Dan White served 5 years and 1 month of his 7-year sentence for shooting and killing two people. After being paroled in the Los Angeles area, where he stayed for a year, White returned to San Francisco. Shortly thereafter, he committed suicide at age 39 (Mathews, 1985).

Diminished Capacity and Criminal Responsibility

Abolishing diminished capacity as a defense in criminal matters was seen by some to have left a hole in the defendant's possible defenses (Weinstock et al., 1996). The only other mental health plea seemed to be not guilty by reason of insanity in states that recognized such a plea. However, if sustained, such a plea could result in the defendant spending the rest of his or her life in a psychiatric institution, whereas a defense of diminished capacity could result in a conviction for a lesser included offense or possibly even an acquittal (Testa & Friedman, 2012).

What did happen in several states is that new terminology replaced diminished capacity as a defense. Defendants now have lists of psychological and other defenses to criminal responsibility, which seems to defy one specific definition (Wilson, 2009). The idea, however, is that if certain conditions are present, the defendant could not form the requisite intent to commit the crime at the time it was perpetrated and is, therefore, not responsible; those conditions could include age, substance abuse, and/or the legal definition of insanity (see Chapter 1.; Texas Penal Code, 2005; Weinstock et al., 1996; Wilson, 2009).

Decision to Bring in a Forensic Psychologist

Whether the defense can be called diminished capacity or any other term the jurisdiction allows, as was seen in *People v. White* (1981), the expertise of a forensic mental health professional is necessary. Law schools provide very little training in mental health, if any, and attorneys are not always aware of their clients' specific psychological or cognitive issues that might be relevant for the defense (Frierson, Boyd, & Harper, 2015). In fact, a recent survey of 492 members of a criminal bar in South Carolina revealed that most thought their law school education regarding mental illness was inadequate (Frierson et al., 2015). Although the study polled only South Carolina attorneys, the individual law schools those attorneys attended were not named and could have represented a cross-section of the country. Further, only attorneys practicing criminal law were participants, and as has been and will be seen, many other specialists and general practitioners have reason to require the services of a forensic psychologist. Insanity is a legal construct, and while attorneys know the law, they depend on the mental health expert to provide a clear picture of their client's psychological status.

The forensic expert has been limited by cases such as *People v. White* (1981) in the scope of permissible testimony, but in working with the attorney can, after a thorough assessment, aid in filling in the psychological information for the legal requirement (Morse, 2000). After the Dan White case, the trend seemed to be to limit any type of diminished capacity defense. Indeed, in 1984, a federal law was enacted that placed the burden on the defendant to show by clear and convincing evidence that the act committed was the "result of a severe mental disease or defect" that prevented the defendant from understanding "the nature and quality" of the acts (Insanity Defense Reform Act, 1984, § 17[a]). In some respects, the need for a forensic mental health expert has increased due to the stricter rules regarding a defendant's plea and the attorney's limited knowledge of the components of mental illness (Frierson et al., 2015).

Type of Case

Most of the time, it is the attorney's decision if and when to bring in a forensic psychologist. As was seen in Chapter 4, the possibility exists in almost all phases of the prosecution of a criminal case (see Figure 4.1). Not only the defense, but also the prosecution and the judge may have questions about competency and request/order a hearing. In a civil matter, the mental health expert might be called upon to provide information on not just competency to participate in a trial, but also competency to contract, state of mind, and intent in specific situations (Perlin, Champine, Dlugacz, & Connell, 2008). For example, minors do not have the capacity to enter into enforceable contracts in most states (Stim, n.d.). However, this is strictly a legal question, and there would be no need to call in an expert to present evidence should a lawsuit ensue; either the individual was over the age of majority when he or she signed the contract or not.

But, as has already been seen in many cases, capacity, intent, and competence in the law may require case-by-case input from an expert in mental health. Contracting, for example, is usually a matter of law regarding the parties, terms, and subject matter requirements; in contrast, the capacity to contract is not based solely on chronological age, but on mental age and psychological fitness as well. While it is settled law that a minor can void a contract under most conditions, whether another individual had the capacity to enter into a contract may be a legal and factual issue that requires the services of a mental health expert (Farnsworth, Sanger, Cohen, Brooks, & Garvin, 2013). As an example, suppose that two parties enter into a contract (we can go back to our pencil example in Chapter 5). The terms are clear that the buyer will pay the seller upon the delivery of the pencils. Upon delivery, the buyer refuses to pay, and the seller sues, attempting to enforce the contract against the buyer. Under the first example of lack of capacity, the buyer states he was only 16 years old when he entered into the contract, and the pencils are not a necessity. In most cases, the seller would immediately lose. However, assume another defense: The buyer asserts he lacked the capacity to contract due to a developmental disability or mental illness. In this case, with no other evidence or just sketchy evidence to go on, the services of a forensic psychologist might be employed to evaluate the cognitive or mental function of the buyer.

Purpose

The attorney may require the services of a forensic psychologist in tort, probate, and family law cases as well. Notwithstanding a court order or request from the other side, it is the right and responsibility of the attorney to decide the purpose for which the psychologist has been hired. While forensic psychologists may be hired for the purpose of jury consulting in criminal and civil matters, witness preparation, or both, the most common reasons for utilizing the services of a forensic psychologist are psychological assessment, including using and interpreting cognitive and psychological tests, and giving expert testimony.

Psychological Assessment

Psychological assessment involves clinical interviewing, gathering of collateral evidence in the form of prior reports and relative and friend interviews, and utilizing valid and reliable psychological testing instruments. In most states, psychological testing must be conducted by a licensed doctoral-level psychologist (Baker, 2016). Psychiatrists, who are medical doctors, do not administer tests and will often refer patients to a psychologist to administer and interpret cognitive and psychological tests (see Chapter 7, Dr. Sammie Williams interview). While most psychologists have vast experience in administering all types of cognitive and psychological instruments, depending upon the purpose, the batteries they administer will usually be limited to the needs of the referral question.

For example, Dr. Richard Delman, the psychologist who testified on behalf of Dan White, administered three psychological tests and came to the conclusion that White was depressed to the extent that he could not have premeditated the killing of two people (*People v. White*, 1981). The record does not specify which tests the psychologist administered, but an educated guess would be that one of them was the Beck Depression Inventory (BDI; 1961), a 21-question self-report that has shown to have validity for measuring symptoms of depression (Beck, Ward, Mendelson, Mock, & Erbaugh, 1961). Because there was also expert testimony that White had average or above-average intelligence, it might be further assumed that a Wechsler Adult Intelligence Scale (WAIS) was administered (see Chapter 7; Cherry, 2017). Currently in its fourth iteration, WAIS provides scores on both achievement and ability levels. It has become "the most frequently administered psychological test" (Cherry, 2017, para. 14). In all likelihood, the psychologist did not administer the original version of the Minnesota Multiphasic Personality Inventory (MMPI), which was published in 1942 (MMPI history, 2017). By the 1970s, it had become the most popular objective measure of personality and psychopathology in use, but it had been normed on a select group of white men in Minnesota, and research and psychological experts called for revisions (Hodges, 2004). Dan White's case spanned 1978 through his 1981 trial, so the 1989 version, MMPI 2, had not yet been released (Groth-Marnat, 1999; MMPI history, 2017). The Rorschach, or inkblot, test had been published in 1922, and by the 1970s it had a uniform scoring system developed by John Exner (1993) (Framingham, 2016). Possibly, the psychologist administered this 10-card projective test and scored it according to Exner's system to come to his testimony regarding White's personality characteristics (Exner, 1993). Although there were and are an infinite number of psychological tests available, the usual battery of a cognitive test and objective and projective personality tests were most likely the basis of Dr. Delman's report (Groth-Marnat, 1999).[1]

Sex offender evaluators such as Dr. Yerke (see Chapter 4) might use the previously mentioned and other instruments as well. When evaluators are assessing sex offenders, they are assessing for risk of recidivism to make release, parole, or probation recommendations. Most states have specific requirements for sex offender evaluators (see, for example, Colorado Standards and Guidelines for the Assessment Evaluation Treatment and Behavioral Monitoring of Adult Sex Offenders; Illinois Sex Offender Evaluation and Treatment Provider Act; and Pennsylvania Sexual Offenders Assessment Board), and some require that standardized tests be administered in the course of the evaluation (see Illinois Sex Offender Evaluation and Treatment Provider Act). California has codified a State-Authorized Risk Assessment Tool for Sexual Offenders Review Committee (SARATSO). Every sex offender required to register in the state is subject to taking at least two tests to help determine the individual's risk of recidivism. By statute, the Static 99R is one of those tests (CA Penal Code § 290.04, 2006). Research has shown that this instrument's predictive validity is good (Lee, Restrepo, Satariano, & Hanson, 2016). The statute also authorizes SARATSO to adopt a dynamic instrument to use in conjunction with the Static 99R, and in 2013, SARATSO adopted the Stable-2007 to help provide more accuracy in assessing (Official Publication, 2017). SARATSO also adopted an instrument to predict risk of future violence, the Level of Service/Case Management Inventory (LS/CMI). While these instruments were adopted solely for use with adult male offenders, the last can be used with females as well. Juvenile offenders are administered another test. As of the beginning of 2017, SARATSO had not found instruments suitable for use with female offenders except the LS/CMI (Official Publication, 2017). Taken together, these three instruments look at unchanging factors such as am individual's history, dynamic factors such as the individual's current situation (e.g., job, family), and risk factors that predict the chances of reoffending. Sex offender evaluators are trained in administering and coding all of these instruments while combining their results with their overall clinical judgment in making their reports.

Child custody evaluators are frequent users of psychological testing instruments and a highly regulated group. The American Association of Matrimonial Lawyers (2011) and much state law guide and direct their work. As was explained in Chapter 5, child custody evaluators are rigidly and specially trained over a period of time and through certain situations. The MMPI 2 is the most frequently used psychological test in child custody cases and can be a valuable tool in assessing overall personalities. In a child custody evaluation, the psychologist will administer the MMPI 2 to both parents and possibly to the child, depending upon the child's age. If the child is old enough, the evaluator might administer the MMPI-A-RF. This adolescent version is shorter and has a slightly lower reading level (Archer, Handel, Ben-Porath, & Tellegen, 2016). If, however, the child is young and cannot take a written test that would result in valid and reliable results, the evaluator may administer the House–Tree–Person (HTP) and/or the Children's Apperception Test (CAT), to name two of the more commonly used children's tests (Buck, 1995; Faust & Ehrich, 2001). Both of these instruments are projective tests designed to elicit unfiltered information from the test takers. The HTP can be used with anyone who can hold a pencil, and the CAT consists of 10 ambiguous animal drawings on separate cards. The latter test was designed to be used with 3- to 10-year-olds.

There are also assessment instruments that were specifically designed to be used for forensic purposes. As mentioned earlier, the Static 99 and Stable-2007 are two that have high validity and reliability. It is probably obvious that due to the use of these instruments in legal settings, their validity is a paramount concern. Specifically, these tests are looking at legal competencies and are by their nature judgmental (Grisso, Borum, Edens, Moye, & Otto, 2003). Although there are dozens of forensic instruments in use at any given time, the Hare Psychopathy Checklist Revised (PCL-R) is in its second edition and is widely used with both male and female adult offenders and forensic populations. This instrument consists of an interview and checklist, should be used only by individuals who have had requisite training, and can take up to 2 hours to administer (DeFabrique, 2011). Although the MMPI 2 and other instruments can be used to test for malingering in forensic populations, the Test of Memory Malingering (TOMM) is another widely used instrument that has predictive validity when used with forensic populations (Weinborn, Orr, Woods, Conover, & Feix, 2003). It is used frequently to look for malingering in cases of competency to stand trial.

Every forensic psychologist has her or his own special battery to be used for a certain purpose, and the more experienced of these professionals are flexible and open to new research regarding newer versions and/or uses for the instruments they adopt (see, for example, Pope, n.d.; Skoler, n.d.). Consideration also needs to be given to the purpose for the testing and the individual being tested (Otto, 2010). As implied by the examples cited previously, the tests used will depend upon whether the issue is child custody, recidivism potential of a sex offender, competency to stand trial, or a myriad of other issues that are commonplace in court proceedings.

Expert Testimony

In 1997, Margaret Hagen, PhD, published *Whores of the Court*, an indictment of expert psychological testimony. She claimed that mental health experts were nothing more than hired guns who usurped the place of the trier of fact in the courts, and she presented well-researched evidence to support her claims. Almost 20 years later, Dr. Hagen (2016) wrote an introduction to the Kindle edition of the book that confirmed her earlier stance, although she recognized that some of the issues of the 1980s and 1990s had been resolved through science. Her examples again are specific and well referenced. While Dr. Hagen's views may be one-sided and a result of her own experience, there is a lesson to be learned for all who would be expert witnesses.[2] *Daubert v. Merrell Dow Pharmaceuticals* (1993) may have opened the gates of the courtroom to expanded admissibility of expert testimony (see Chapter 5), but the presentation still should not go beyond the science (Federal Rule of Evidence 702; Schweitzer & Saks, 2009). The Federal Rules of Evidence and ethical considerations of both professions require that the jury not be misled in any way (ABA Model Rules, 2002; American Psychological Association, 2017). Expert testimony is a two-step process: Once admitted, the weight given to it can be determinative of a jury decision, and jurors are swayed by judges' admissibility decisions and experts' long lists of credentials (Schweitzer & Saks, 2009). Not only does the expert have the duty to refrain from testifying beyond the scope of his or her knowledge, but the attorney also needs to choose the expert carefully (Hamza, 2016).

As was the case in the trial of Dan White, psychological testing results often become part of the case record and are introduced by the forensic psychologist who administered and interpreted the tests.

They most likely are the science to which Hagen (2016) was referring. The attorneys interviewed in this chapter share similar opinions about the experts with whom they consult and bring into their cases. Although they do not explicitly use the word, both attorneys hire experts with whom they can establish rapport. Attorneys also need to have a basic understanding of the psychometric instruments the experts use, just as the experts need to have a basic understanding of the law or laws at issue (Hamza, 2016). When both parties are aware of their roles and follow the rules of the court and their ethical codes, the expert and the attorney can become a strong, persuasive, and cohesive team.

Recognizing the Similarities and Differences

Part of becoming a team is recognizing and acknowledging similarities and differences. Lawyers and psychologists have ethical codes, practice codes within which they operate, a focus of inquiry, and facts on which they base that focus.

Ethical Codes

The American Bar Association has published Model Rules of Professional Conduct (2002), and almost all states have based their own ethical codes for attorneys on those rules.[3] The Model Rules are aspirational rather than enforceable, but attorneys are subject to their own state codes and rules regarding ethical behavior, which are enforceable. Forensic psychologists are first clinicians who are subject to the enforceable standards of the American Psychological Association's (2017) *Ethical Principles of Psychologists and Code of Conduct* (*EPPCC*). While the five ethical principles are aspirational, the standards that follow are enforceable (American Psychological Association, 2017). Forensic psychologists also operate with knowledge of the aspirational goals of the *Specialty Guidelines for Forensic Psychology* (American Psychological Association, 2013).

Attorneys and forensic psychologists, then, have two sets of ethical guidelines that are both aspirational and enforceable. Within those principles, standards, rules, and guidelines are both similarities and conflicts. Both professions need to avoid conflicts of interest, maintain confidentiality, and not act outside their scope of competence (ABA Model Rules, 2002; American Psychological Association, 2017). They owe a fiduciary duty to their clients, but the attorney is an advocate (ABA Model Rules, 2002). The forensic psychologist, however, is not an advocate. He or she is an objective evaluator, and the individual with whom this professional may have the most contact is probably not the client (American Psychological Association, 2013).

The forensic practitioners, however, might have one ethical dilemma that attorneys do not face. As will be seen in *Jaffee v. Redmond*, practitioners' ethical standards may conflict with the law. The *Specialty Guidelines for Forensic Psychology*, in agreement with the *EPPCC* (2017), caution about conflicts with legal authority. Guideline 7.01 advises the forensic psychologist to resolve the conflict "in accordance with the *EPPCC*." If a conflict cannot be resolved, the forensic practitioner may follow the law but not to the extent that anyone's human rights might be violated.

Laws and the DSM

While attorneys may not be able to quote the wording of every law for every topic, they do know what laws they need and where to find them. They gather all available evidence and match the facts of their case with the law that applies. This is how attorneys narrow the issues for trial or a possible earlier resolution of their case. When psychologists have a case referred, they have an express or implied, broad or narrow referral question and the *Diagnostic and Statistical Manual of Mental Disorders* (*DSM-5*; American Psychiatric Association, 2013). After amassing their evidence by way of testing, interviewing, and reviewing records, they come to the relevant facts and match those facts to the appropriate criteria for the disorder in the *DSM*. Forensic psychologists, depending upon the circumstances, may have access to the relevant law as well and be able to apply their knowledge to it. Recall Dr. James Earnest's interview in Chapter 3. As a forensic psychologist working for the county, he is familiar with the facts that the court wants to know about a particular individual and the law that will be applied. California Welfare and Institutions Code §5150 allows for involuntary confinement if, among other things, an individual is "gravely disabled." Dr. Earnest will report all those facts about the individual so that the court can make the legal determination (Shelton, Goldner, & Henry, 2016).

Issues And Referral Question

As has been discussed in previous chapters and illustrated in the example cases, attorneys gather their information so as to address and possibly narrow the issues before the court. Courts will address only issues that are put in writing and raised by the parties involved in the case (see, for example, *People v. White*, 1981). Whether the case is criminal or civil, juvenile or family, it is up to the parties involved to tell the court what they want. The forensic psychologist is called upon to help or just clarify those issues before the court. The psychologist, then, addresses the referral question. What does the client want to know? The referral question may go to the main issue in the case, such as a child custody dispute. The attorney will tell the court why it is in the child's best interest to be in the custody of his or her client and do so with evidence partially provided by the child custody evaluator. However, the evaluator's referral question will not ask for the legal conclusion, it will ask for an evaluation of all the parties so that the determination can be made as to what custody arrangement is in the best interest of the child.

The forensic psychologist's referral question may be collateral to the case. A criminal defense attorney whose client is on trial for burglary, for example, may find that the client is most uncooperative in the planning of the case. The client may have a partial alibi or other defense to the actual crime, but the attorney cannot get enough information to plan the trial strategy. Although his or her role does not speak to whether the client committed the burglary, a forensic psychologist might be called in to evaluate the client's understanding of the nature of the legal proceedings and to determine whether the defendant understands and can be of aid to the attorney in his or her own defense. After the evaluation, the court can determine from the information if, according to the law, the defendant is competent to stand trial.

Another difference in the roles of the attorney and the forensic psychologist is the basis of their professions. Attorneys have a burden of proof. If the case is criminal, the burden is beyond a reasonable doubt, and the evidence should be such that the jury cannot have a reasonable doubt as to what the verdict should be. Civil cases usually require a preponderance of the evidence. Evidence is offered as proof of the matter (Federal Rules of Evidence 103, 801). In the law, although not absolute, this is enough proof. In psychology, the term used is "probability." Psychologists can only falsify, not prove, their theories (Popper, 2002). They usually do this by using the scientific method of deductive reasoning, which relies on probability. Researchers develop a theory; from the theory, they develop a hypothesis. If the hypothesis is not falsified during the testing, it becomes a probability that in some circumstances can be generalized (Popper, 2002). Depending on the standard set, the probability could be 95% or higher, but it is not scientific proof.

The law also uses both inductive and deductive reasoning. The attorney begins with the law and matches it to the facts of the case. When the facts and the law do not quite match, the attorney deduces the issue. That issue is then presented to the court for resolution, and the resolution could be a new application of a law that can eventually be applied to other cases. Thus, the inductive process is basically used at the beginning of legal analysis to help form a general rule; the result then moves into the deductive process by applying it to a fact situation. And subsequently evolves into a new rule. In fact, in legal analysis, the process of inductive and deductive reasoning usage becomes almost circular (Aldisert, 1989). The forensic psychologist, as an advisor or expert, is actually part of the attorney's evidence—that part of the evidence that requires expert advice or opinion as the offer of proof. The forensic psychologist then can speak and/or attest to the probability of a scientifically tested opinion (Figure 8.1).

SPOTLIGHT ON CASES

A third party, the therapist or clinician, might also enter into the picture. Just as there might be some confusion or blurring between the role of the attorney and the role of the forensic psychologist, so there might also be an issue requiring clarification between the forensic psychologist and the therapist or clinician in a legal setting. As seen in Chapter 3, the mindset and the processes used are different

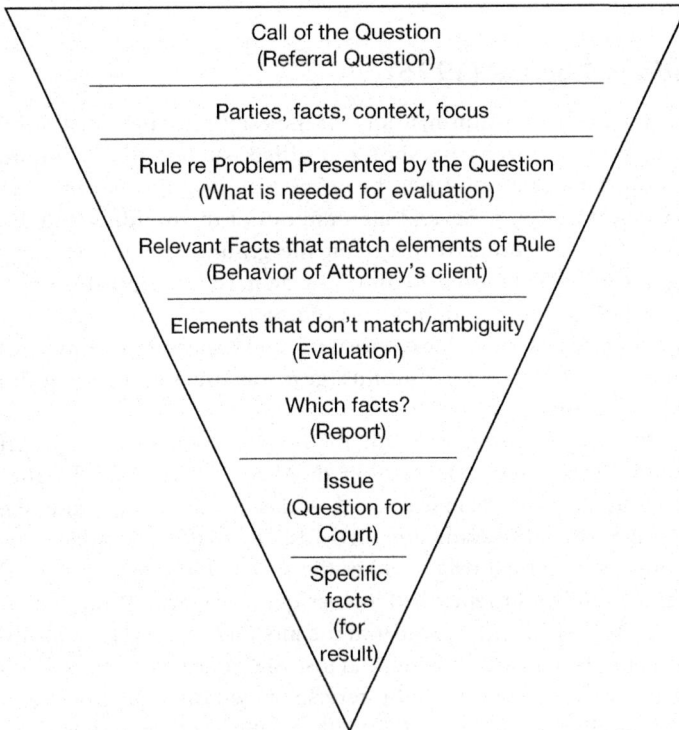

Call of the Question
(Referral Question)

Parties, facts, context, focus

Rule re Problem Presented by the Question
(What is needed for evaluation)

Relevant Facts that match elements of Rule
(Behavior of Attorney's client)

Elements that don't match/ambiguity
(Evaluation)

Which facts?
(Report)

Issue
(Question for
Court)

Specific
facts
(for
result)

Teamwork: Issue Recognition and Resolution
1. Attorney/court presents question
   Psychologist addresses referral question
2. Attorney relies on statutory/case law
   Psychologist relies on *DSM*
3. Attorney narrows facts to ambiguity
   Psychologist evaluates to recommendation
4. Court/jury weigh facts, evaluation, law
   Facts + instructions = result

FIGURE 8.1 Finding and defining the issue. Thinking like a lawyer. (For the forensic psychologist.)

for these professionals, as are some ethical considerations. When the issues get to court, the legal system also has a say in the resolution. The United States (U.S.) Supreme Court case that follows illustrates some of the issues.

Jaffee v. Redmond (1996)

Facts: Jaffee is the administrator of the estate of Allen. Redmond was a police officer who shot and killed Allen while Redmond was on duty. Redmond had been called to an altercation at an apartment building. Several men ran out of the building and did not obey the command to get on the ground. Allen was carrying a knife and ignored Redmond's demand to drop the knife. Redmond said she thought he was going to use it to stab another man, and the situation was threatening. Witnesses (members of Allen's family) stated Redmond's gun was drawn and Allen did not have a weapon.

Procedure: Jaffee filed suit in Illinois Federal District Court for wrongful death and violation of Allen's constitutional rights. Redmond had seen a clinical social worker about 50 times after the shooting, and Jaffee wanted the records. The trial judge ordered the records to be turned over. Neither the social worker nor Redmond would comply and refused to answer questions or said they could not remember. The trial judge told the jury there was no legal justification for the refusal and Redmond lost. She appealed to the Seventh Circuit Court of Appeals, and it reversed based on its interpretation of Federal Rule of Evidence (FRE) 501 and the fact that all states have a law granting a privilege of confidentiality to the patient–therapist relationship. Because the question goes to the interpretation of FRE 501, and because there are conflict and controversy about this question, the U.S. Supreme Court agreed to hear the case on the one issue.

Issue: Does the Federal Rule of Evidence protect the therapist–patient relationship?

Holding: Since Illinois state law protects the privilege and FRE 501 gives a general privilege of confidentiality and makes state law paramount, FRE 501 protects the interest of the client.

Judgment: Affirmed for Redmond.

FOCUS ON CAREERS

While what follows should in no way be interpreted as an endorsement to attend law school, there are several programs that grant a JD/PhD or PsyD at the end of several years of study. Knowing that I am an attorney and have a PhD in psychology, many students have come to me over the years asking if I thought they should go to law school. My advice is always the same. As would any lawyer, I start by asking a question: Do you want to practice law? If the answer is an unequivocal and exclusive "yes," I tell them to go to law school. The psychology background will be helpful in practice. If the response is something like what I hear more frequently, "Well, I don't know; I just know I like them both," I explain they cannot be both at the same time. They are both professions, and each has its own hat to wear (Strasburger, Gutheil, & Brodsky, 1997). Common sense tells us we can wear only one hat at a time. So, when reading the attorney interviews, keep in mind that although both have been in practice for decades and learned a lot about psychology during the course of their careers, neither would attempt to act in the place of a forensic psychologist.

STEPHAN DESALES, ESQ.

Stephan DeSales, Esq., is a criminal law defense attorney who is licensed to practice in several states and in front of the U.S. Supreme Court. His original career goal included a life in politics. However, after graduating from the University of Notre Dame Law School and passing the California State Bar Exam, he went to work in the Los Angeles County District Attorney's office. After a couple of years, Mr. DeSales went into private practice doing defense work. Although he began practicing law over 40 years ago, Mr. DeSales cannot remember a time when criminal defense

(*continued*)

(continued)

attorneys did not utilize the services of forensic psychologists for various purposes during the course of a criminal trial.

With over 250 trials and innumerable cases that were resolved before trial behind him, Mr. DeSales is clear about the types of services he needs from forensic psychologists. He looks at those services as a strong "weapon in the arsenal" of evidence he can utilize for his clients. First, he considers whether his client is factually and legally not guilty (i.e., the client was not present at the crime). If this is the case, it would be rare for him to utilize the services of a forensic psychologist. Since the state needs to prove the defendant guilty beyond a reasonable doubt in a criminal trial, Mr. DeSales would not usually have the need for providing technical defenses. However, if the case requires technical defenses, and if the facts presented warrant it, he may hire a forensic psychologist to provide several services.

Among the issues specifically addressed by the forensic psychologists he has hired have been competency to stand trial, expert testimony on eyewitness testimony, and jury consulting. Regarding competency to stand trial, Mr. DeSales has been in situations where he, the prosecutor, or the judge might suspect the defendant is not competent to stand trial (see Chapter 4). When this happens, a forensic psychologist is hired to evaluate the individual and his or her ability to understand the nature of the proceedings against him or her (CA Penal Code § 1368). At any time during the proceedings, if Mr. DeSales is the one asking for the services of a forensic psychologist, if at all possible he chooses carefully from several with whom he has worked. He takes into account not only their professional skill regarding reporting on the particular issue, but also their personalities, ability to relate to people, and any prior dealings with the judge and the specific court. Recently, in fact, he interviewed and hired a forensic psychologist with whom he had no prior dealings to help evaluate his client's competency. The client's

(continued)

(*continued*)

first language was Spanish, and Mr. DeSales wanted a Spanish-speaking evaluator to conduct the evaluation.

The expert he called upon to testify as to the reliability of eyewitness testimony was recruited for the trial of an accused sex offender. In this case, the offender was facing 11 counts of sex with a minor. The minor involved was the 17-year-old niece of the defendant's girlfriend, who was the eyewitness for the prosecution. The expert not only had the expertise to discuss the historical unreliability of eyewitness testimony, but also pointed out attributes of the State's eyewitness that allowed the defense to cross-examine and minimize her testimony and impact the jury's decision.

Just as an experienced forensic psychologist understands how the law works constitutionally, statutorily, and as precedent from the cases, an experienced criminal defense attorney recognizes, understands, and knows how to use the psychological terminology applicable in a given fact situation. In discussing his employment of forensic psychologists, Mr. DeSales refers to the changing legal terminology and factual requirements with which he and his experts must contend. One example is the term "diminished capacity," which, prior to 1982 in California (and still in federal courts and some states), was a mitigating defense for various criminal acts, allowing for conviction of a lesser act or lighter sentencing if proven (CA Penal Code § 25, 1982; *People v. White*, 1981; Testa & Friedman, 2012). Since California abolished diminished capacity as a defense, when circumstances permit, the defense is now criminal responsibility. It is the attorney's job to know the law, but the attorney relies on the forensic psychologist to determine whether the evaluation of the client meets the legal standards. Further, if the report is not favorable to the defense, there is no obligation to use it. As a collateral matter, this fact helps ensure the objectivity and professionalism of the forensic evaluator (American Psychological Association, 2013).

(*continued*)

(*continued*)

MICHAEL FISHER, ESQ.

Michael Fisher, Esq., is a certified family law attorney in California who had a previous career as a math teacher in the state of Washington. Since 1988, when he joined an existing small practice, he has been practicing family law. In 1994, he achieved his certification through the California State Bar Board of Legal Specialization, and he has been recognized by *Super Lawyers Magazine* as a super lawyer five times between 2004 and 2016.

Becoming a Certified Family Law Specialist in California is a year-long process. Prior to taking an examination, the applicant must have been a practicing attorney for 5 years, with at least 25% of the practice in family law. Three attorneys or judges must write letters of recommendation that include evaluations of the attorney's work. California attorneys need 25 hours of continuing education every 3 years; certified specialists must report 36 hours. After having taken and passed the certification exam, the remainder of the application process requires that the attorney have been the principal attorney in at least four of five requirements: 20 contested family law hearings, five hearings or trials of at least 3 hours in length and involving witnesses, 30 negotiated judgments or settlements, 30 stipulated family law orders, and three family appeals. The requirements also list 12 areas of family law in which the attorney had to participate, including the psychological and counseling aspects of family law.[4]

Since California has been a no-fault dissolution state since 1970 and has allowed bifurcation since 1992, most of the trials that Mr. Fisher has been involved in have had to do with the financial aspects of dissolution or the terms of a contract. The vast majority of his cases were eventually settled, but one continued for 8 years before the economics of the case were finally apportioned.

As does Stephan DeSales, Michael Fisher utilizes the services of a forensic psychologist for several different reasons, although

(*continued*)

(*continued*)

he says custody issues are the most common. In California, custody evaluations are also called 730 evaluations, as they are authorized by § 730 of the California Evidence Code. The code section allows for the appointment and testimony of experts, usually in child custody conflicts. Since the court makes these orders on its own motion, Mr. Fisher may not have his choice of evaluators. He does, however, have the right to object if he has grounds. When asked what he does if the evaluation is unfavorable to his client, his response is both interesting and responsible: He often consults with another forensic psychologist to learn if there are ways to combat the negativity. Sometimes this entails the psychologist meeting his client, and sometimes even that report is less than he had hoped for.

However, when this happens, Mr. Fisher at least has a framework for helping his client reach a compromise regarding the custody or visitation arrangement at issue. Sometimes, he consults a forensic psychologist prior to the investigatory phase to help frame the case, discuss problematic issues, or just figure out how to approach a particular case. This person will always be an individual with whom he has worked before, and he may even have the psychologist meet his client. He recalls a case involving a client who was a recovering heroin addict. She was sober when she hired Mr. Fisher, but he wanted more information, so he employed the forensic consultant to help him determine his client's potential for recidivism and to meet with the client to help her understand what the court would be looking for.

One of the more common causes for parents losing custody is addiction, usually to drugs or alcohol, although Mr. Fisher did have a client whose addiction was viewing pornography. One of the saddest cases he was involved in was a dissolution caused by the husband's impending gender transition. The wife was deeply religious and immediately filed for divorce and sole custody of their children. Against Mr. Fisher's advice, the husband refused to go to counseling or discuss the matter with

(*continued*)

(*continued*)

his children. At some point during the lengthy negotiations and various hearings, the father seemed to have given up and disappeared. Michael Fisher says that although this happened many years ago, he still thinks about that family and hopes they all did eventually get counseling and share their lives.

After a very successful career, Mr. Fisher now calls himself retired from active practice. He limits his professional time to family law mediation, a time- and money-saving way to achieve a realistic compromised dissolution settlement.

IN THE NEWS

In November 2016, Brandon Colbert allegedly shot and killed a mother and her young daughter. After his arrest, he had multiple court hearings and evaluations as to his mental competency while he remained in jail. The relevance of his case to this chapter is that not only was Colbert's mental competency scrutinized, but during these hearings he also acted as his own attorney. By May 30, 2017, he was found to be incompetent to stand trial and was committed for no less than 90 days. If he is restored to competency to stand trial, according to the prosecutor, he will have to undergo another evaluation to determine if he is competent to be his own attorney (Queally, 2017). The roles here would be so confusing as to make one wonder how justice can be served. Colbert would be both the defendant and the attorney for the defense.

SUMMARY

This chapter compared and contrasted the roles of the forensic psychologist and the lawyer as well as distinguished the role of the therapist. The comparison between the two disciplines involved looking at some of the ethics and the analytical reasoning required of the practitioners The attorney was shown to be the chief strategist, while the forensic psychologist uses specialized knowledge to respond to the attorney's referral question. In the process, the forensic psychologist uses interviewing techniques and research, and has numerous valid and reliable psychological tests available to administer and interpret.

The example cases were chosen to illustrate how expert psychological testimony can contribute to changing the law (*People v. White*, 1981) and differentiating the responsibility/duty of the forensic psychologist and the therapist (*Jaffee v. Redmond*, 1996). To change the perspective from that of the forensic practitioner, two attorneys who utilize the services of forensic psychologists were profiled. Since they practice two very different specialties, criminal law and family law, their experiences and perspectives were also quite different and highly educational.

DISCUSSION QUESTIONS

1. Psychopathy is defined in the *DSM-5* (American Psychiatric Association, 2013) as antisocial personality disorder. Individuals with antisocial personality disorder are considered mentally ill. Their behavior shows disregard for the rights of others, no remorse for their behavior, and incessant lying, among other traits (Strickland, Drislane, Lucy, Krueger, & Patrick, 2013). Not all criminals are psychopaths, and not all psychopaths are criminals. Discuss your thoughts about psychopaths claiming a diminished capacity or diminished actuality defense to a criminal accusation (Weinstock et al., 1996).

2. Discuss your understanding of the relative importance of the interview and use of testing instruments in forensic evaluations. Do you think either is more important in a clinical interview?

3. Can the decisions in *Jaffee v. Redmond* (1996) and *Mathews v. Harris* (2017) be reconciled? If so, what is the explanation?

NOTES

1. For a complete list and explanations of available psychological tests, the *Mental Measurements Yearbook* (MMY; Buros Center for Testing) is published every 3 years. As of 2017, the current edition is the *Twentieth Mental Measurements Yearbook*. All tests that appear in the MMY must be available, be published in English, and include enough information so that the test can be reviewed. Each test is reviewed by two professionals whose references are listed. Each test appears in only one MMY unless it is has been completely revised and/or is in much wider usage than its previous appearance. More information is available at http://buros.org/mental-measurements-yearbook.
2. Introduction to 1997 edition of *Whores of the Court.*
3. As of May 30, 2017, California was still the only state whose Rules of Professional Conduct were not based on the ABA Model. However, the Commission for the Revision of the Rules of Professional Conduct of the State Bar of California had submitted amendments to the California Supreme Court and was awaiting a final decision.
4. Information from State Bar of California website: http://www.calbar.ca.gov/Attorneys/Legal-Specialization/Legal-Specialty-Areas/Family-Law

REFERENCES

ABA Model Rules of Professional Conduct. (2002). *American Bar Association.* Retrieved from https://www.law.cornell.edu/ethics/aba

Aldisert, R. J. (1989). *Logic for lawyers: A guide to clear legal thinking.* New York, NY: Clark Boardman.

American Association of Matrimonial Lawyers. (2011). *Child custody evaluation standards.* Retrieved from http://aaml.org/library/publications/child-custody-evaluation-standards-doc

American Psychiatric Association. (2013). *Diagnostic and statistical manual of mental disorders* (5th ed.). Washington, DC: Author.

American Psychological Association. (2013). Specialty guidelines for forensic psychology. *American Psychologist, 68*(1), 7–19. doi:10.1037/a0029889).

American Psychological Association. (2017). *Ethical principles of psychologists and code of conduct.* Washington, DC: Author. Retrieved from http://www.apa.org/ethics/code/ethics-code-2017.pdf

Archer, R. P., Handel, R. W., Ben-Porath, Y. S., & Tellegen, A. (2016). *Minnesota Multiphasic Personality Inventory-Adolescent-Restructure Form (MMPI-A-RF)*. Retrieved from http://www.pearsonclinical.com/psychology/products/100001762/minnesota-multiphasic-personality-inventoryadolescent-restructured-form-mmpi-a-rf.html

Baker, D. (2016, February). *Who can conduct testing? What do state practice acts say?* Presented at APA Practice State Leadership Conference, Washington, DC.

Beck, A. T., Ward, C. H., Mendelson, M., Mock, J., & Erbaugh, J. (1961). An inventory for measuring depression. *Archives of General Psychiatry, 4*, 561–571.

Buck, J. N. (1995). *House–tree–person projective drawing technique: Manual and interpretive guide*. Torrance, CA: WPS.

Calcagno, W. (1991). Instructions to the jury. In K. W. Salter (Ed.), *The trial of Dan White*. Retrieved from http://www.famous-trials.com/danwhite/590-juryinstructions

California Penal Code §§ 25, 187, 192, 290.04.

California Welfare & Institutions Code § 5150, Lanterman Petris Short Act (1972).

Cherry, K. (2017). The Wechsler Adult Intelligence Scale: History and use of the WAIS. *Verywell*. Retrieved from https://www.verywell.com/the-wechsler-adult-intelligence-scale-2795283

DeFabrique, N. (2011). Hare psychopathy checklist. In *Encyclopedia of clinical neuropsychology* (pp. 1210–1211). New York, NY: Springer.

Exner, J. E. (1993). *The Rorschach: A comprehensive system. Volume 1: Basic foundations* (3rd ed.). New York, NY: Wiley.

Farnsworth, E. A., Sanger, C., Cohen, N. B., Brooks, R. R. W., & Garvin, L. T. (2013). *Contracts cases and materials* (8th ed.). Kennewick, WA: Foundation Press.

Faust, J., & Ehrich, S. (2001). Children's Apperception Test (C.A.T.). In W. I. Dorfman & M. Hersen (Eds.), *Understanding psychological assessment: Perspectives on individual differences*. Boston, MA: Springer.

Framingham, J. (2016). Rorschach inkblot test. *Psych Central*. Retrieved from https://psychcentral.com/lib/rorschach-inkblot-test/

Frierson, R. L., Boyd, M. S., & Harper, A. (2015). Mental illness and mental health defenses: Perceptions of the criminal bar. *Journal of the American Academy of Psychiatry & the Law, 43*(4), 483–491.

Grisso, T., Borum, R., Edens, J. F., Moye, J., & Otto, R. K. (2003). *Evaluating competencies: Forensic assessments and instruments* (2nd ed.). New York, NY: Springer.

Groth-Marnat, G. (1999). *Handbook of psychological assessment* (3rd ed.). New York, NY: Wiley.

Hagen, M. A. (1997, 2016). *Whores of the court* [Kindle edition]. New York, NY: HarperCollins.

Hamza, M. Z. (2016). *The roles of forensic mental health experts in the legal system: What practitioners of law may need to know.* Retrieved from http://www.voiceforthedefenseonline.com/story/roles-forensic-mental-health-experts-legal-system-what-practitioners-law-may-need-know

Hodges, P. (2004). *The MMPI 1 & 2.* Unpublished work.

Insanity Defense Reform Act of 1984. 18 U.S.C. 17.

Jaffee v. Redmond 518 U.S. 1 (1996).

Krassner, P. (2011). Behind the infamous Twinkie defense. *Huffington Post.* Retrieved from http://www.huffingtonpost.com/paul-krassner/behind-the-infamous-twink_b_148474.html

Lee, S. C., Restrepo, A., Satariano, A., & Hanson, R. K. (2016). *The predictive validity of Static-99R for sexual offenders in California.* Retrieved from http://www.saratso.org/docs/ThePredictiveValidity_of_Static-99R_forSexualOffenders_inCalifornia-2016v1.pdf

Linder, D. O. (n.d.-a). The trial of Dan White: Selected testimony. *Famous Trials.* Retrieved from http://www.famous-trials.com/danwhite/597-testimony

Linder, D. O. (n.d.-b) The trial of Dan White: The testimony of Dr. Martin Blinder. Retrieved from http://www.famous-trials.com/danwhite/601-Llindertestimony

Mathews, J. (1985, October 22). Dan White commits suicide. *Washington Post.* Retrieved from https://www.washingtonpost.com/archive/politics/1985/10/22/dan-white-commits-suicide/590322ca-f461-4a98-9c5f-348648f7ac66/?utm_term=.e92bbc21a09d

MMPI history. (2017). *A brief history of the MMPI instruments.* University of Minnesota Press. Retrieved from https://www.upress.umn.edu/test-division/bibliography/mmpi-history

Morse, S. J. (2000). Rationality and responsibility. *Southern California Law Review, 74,* 251–268.

Official publication of the SARATSO review and training committee. (2017). *Sex offender risk assessment in California.* Retrieved from http://www.saratso.org/docs/RA_summary_for_judges_attys_rev_1-3-17.pdf

Otto, R. K. (2010). Forensic assessment instruments and techniques [Abstract]. *Mental Health Law & Policy Faculty Publications.* Retrieved from http://scholarcommons.usf.edu/mhlp_facpub/154/

People v. White 117 Cal.APP 3d 270. (1981, March 25). Retrieved from http://www.famous-trials.com/danwhite/596-peoplevwhite

Perlin, M. L., Champine, P. R., Dlugacz, H. A., & Connell, M. (2008). *Competence in the law.* Hoboken, NJ: Wiley.

Pope, K. S. (n.d.). Psychological assessment: Clinical and forensic. *Articles, Research, & Resources in Psychology*. Retrieved from https://kspope.com/assess/malinger.php

Popper, K. (2002). *The logic of scientific discovery*. New York, NY: Routledge.

Queally, J. (2017, May 30). In court, baffling claims. *Los Angeles Times*. Retrieved from http://www.latimes.com/local/lanow/la-me-long-beach-murder-mental-illness-20170512-story.html

Schweitzer, N. J., & Saks, M. J. (2009). The gatekeeper effect: The impact of judges' admissibility decisions on the persuasiveness of expert testimony. *Psychology, Public Policy & Law, 15*(1), 1–18.

Shelton, S., Goldner, J. A., & Henry, J. (2016). Psychologist in the legal system: Merging and avoiding collisions at the intersection of psychology and law. *Register Report*. Retrieved from https://www.nationalregister.org/pub/the-national-register-report-pub/the-register-report-fall-2016/psychologists-in-the-legal-system-merging-and-avoiding-collisions-at-the-intersection-of-psychology-and-law/

Skoler, G. (n.d.). *Psychological tests list*. Retrieved from http://www.clinicalandforensicpsychology.com/DrGlenSkoler/Psychological_Tests_List.html

Stim, R. (n.d.). Who lacks the capacity to contract? *Nolo*. Retrieved from http://www.nolo.com/legal-encyclopedia/lack-capacity-to-contract-32647.html

Strasburger, L. H., Gutheil, T. G., & Brodsky, A. (1997). On wearing two hats: Role conflict in serving as both psychotherapist and expert witness. *American Journal of Psychiatry, 154*(4), 448–456.

Strickland, C. M., Drislane, L. E., Lucy, M., Krueger, R. F., & Patrick, C. J. (2013). Characterizing psychopathy using *DSM-5* personality traits. *Assessment, 20*(3), 327–338.

Testa, M., & Friedman, S. H. (2012). Diminished capacity. *Journal of the American Academy of Psychiatry and the Law, 40*(4), 567–569.

Texas Penal Code. (2005). *Chapter 8. General defenses to criminal responsibility*. Retrieved from http://www.texas-statutes.com/penal-code/chapter-8-general-defenses-to-criminal-responsibility

Weinborn, M., Orr, T., Woods, S. P., Conover, E., & Feix, J. (2003). A validation of the test of memory malingering in a forensic setting. *Journal of Clinical and Experimental Neuropsychology, 25*(7), 979–990.

Weinstock, R., Leong, G. B., & Silva, J. A. (1996). California's diminished capacity defense: Evolution and transformation. *Bulletin of the American Academy of Psychiatry & the Law, 24*(3), 347–366.

Wilson, S. (2009). Criminal responsibility. *Psychiatry, 8*(12), 473–475.

The Growing Future of Forensic Psychology

OVERVIEW

Since 1962, when the United States (U.S.) Supreme Court decided that psychologists could testify as experts in court, opportunity in the field of forensic psychology has continued to expand (*Jenkins v. United States*). If forensic psychology is psychology for any legal purpose, no volume could do justice to the various areas of psychology and the law in which forensic psychologists have the opportunity to work. The goal of the interviews, cases, and other examples in this book was to provide an introduction to the broad spectrum of possibilities—from full- or part-time employment in the courts, to independent legal-based subspecialties, to research and academia. However, some of the current opportunities and their future applications were not addressed. This chapter fills in some of those areas. However, since every day seems to bring about more opportunities for forensic psychologists, the chapter should not be considered all inclusive.

Statistics are clear that forensic psychologists are high earners in the psychology world and in great demand (Bureau of Labor Statistics, 2016). Some areas do not fit neatly into particular court divisions, however, so they are explored here to help illustrate the future of forensic psychology. As was seen in *Elonis v. United States* (2015) and *Romano v. Steelcase* (2010), the development of **social media** has created another area for the work of forensic psychologists—whether the work is evaluation, research, or expertise about human behavior to educate a jury, forensic psychologists are being hired. Advances in **neurotechnology** have opened up even more opportunities for forensic psychologists to provide testimony.

Several specific law-related areas of psychology are addressed as areas of opportunity. **Law enforcement**, **gangs**, **correctional psychology**, and the study of **terrorism/violence** are all areas of interest for forensic psychologists and can be viewed as subspecialties of forensic psychology. A law enforcement entity can be anything from the local police station, to a district attorney's office, to any one of the federal agencies, including the Federal Bureau of Investigation (FBI), Bureau of Alcohol, Tobacco, and Firearms (ATF), and Immigration and Customs Enforcement (ICE), all of which have very high media profiles. References to some of the forensic psychologists who were interviewed bring the overview full circle, as do the cases and topical news stories.

HOW IT WORKS

American Psychological Association and Forensic Psychology

Although it recognized forensic psychology as a specialty in 2001, as of 2017 no academic forensic program has been accredited by the American Psychological Association (APA, 2017a). For various but unknown reasons, applications have been rejected, and as a result some programs are no longer operating to grant the forensic psychology doctorate. The APA accredits only doctoral-level programs, and those seem to be limited to mostly clinical, education, and counseling specialties (Marker, 2017). There are, however, forensic psychology certificates or specializations available at various institutions whose clinical programs are APA accredited. Most, if not all, programs require a yearlong predoctoral internship before the granting of a degree. Unfortunately, many internship opportunities accept only students who attend an APA-accredited program, making it difficult for a forensic psychology student to achieve his or her career goals. If a student wants a career with any of the federal agencies, in a federal prison, or in a veterans' hospital or with the Veterans Administration, an alternative is to attend an APA-accredited clinical program that offers either a certificate or specialization in forensic psychology. However, for some individuals, the forensic psychology degree is the main reason they put so many years into attaining a doctoral degree, and they want the psycholegal experience that the program offers.

An alternative would be to work toward a combined psychology doctoral and law degree; these programs are few and far between, however, and take upwards of 6 years to complete. Pure forensic and clinical forensic doctoral programs still do exist, and the graduates are quickly finding jobs in the field with salaries higher than those of general psychology graduates. When a student has a clear picture of his or her future career, making the choice becomes much easier. Further, previous work experience, location, and practicum placements do matter, as do performance and perseverance. Everyone involved, from academics to legal professionals, seem to agree that the need and positions for forensic psychologists are on the rise. One state, California, has its own internship match program, but cannot guarantee a student will be eligible for licensure in another state (CAPIC, 2017). At some point, the APA could rethink what seems to be almost automatic rejection of forensic psychology program applications, as the need is consistently expanding.

Areas of Opportunity

As the opportunities for forensic psychologists increase, forensic psychology is breeding a discipline of subspecialties. The potential is endless for those who are looking for new pathways in legal or court-related psychology. A few of those areas are described next and offer research, practice, and academic pathways.

Social Media

The development of social media has contributed to much litigation and an even greater need for psychological expertise in the courts. Earlier chapters gave examples of *Elonis v. United States* (2015), *Romano v. Steelcase* (2010), and two suicide-related cases that ended up in the courts due to the defendants' use of social media. In addition to the cases mentioned, social media have played key roles in cases dealing with sex trafficking, vehicular manslaughter, marital infidelity, and even traffic violations.

In *United States v. Anderson* (2012), Anderson had solicited minors for sex through social media. He was eventually caught, tried, and convicted because a 13-year-old finally told her mother about the meetings. The mother went to the authorities, who were able to arrest, try, and convict him after the mother, in her daughter's name, made a date to meet with Anderson.

Eighteen-year-old Nicole Hoffman was driving under the influence of marijuana and alcohol while texting and talking on her cell phone. She had two passengers in her car, one of whom died when she crashed. Before the accident, she had been arrested twice for "alcohol-related offenses" and posted pictures of herself with alcohol on social media. She was sentenced to 9 years in prison, with the court saying that her online postings were one of the aggravating factors that led to her long sentence (*Hoffman v. State,* 2012).

White v. White (2001) was a family law case involving a bitter custody battle. The wife found a letter on the family computer from the husband's girlfriend. The husband wanted the letter suppressed; he claimed its admission was an invasion of his privacy. Its admission could negatively affect his bid for custody of his children. The court, however, admitted the letter, saying there was no privacy once the item was actually stored on a family computer.

Finally, *People v. Spriggs* (2014) started out in traffic court. California has a law against using a handheld telephone and/or texting while driving (CVC 23123 (a)). Mr. Spriggs was using his cell phone for its Global Positioning System (GPS) capability, looking for an alternative route to the stalled traffic he was in. He was ordered to pay $165 fine in traffic court. He appealed to the superior court, which confirmed the fine, and Spriggs then appealed to the state appeals court based on the wording of the statute. The statute stated that there could be no communication on a phone unless it was hands free. The appeals court reversed the finding of the two lower courts, saying that Mr. Spriggs was not communicating, but merely checking a route.

Dozens more cases could be cited, including those involving cyberbullying, identity theft, various Internet scams, and more; they are criminal and civil and family and First Amendment cases. Participating in the cases or researching the phenomenon of social media in the courts represents both the present and the future for interested forensic psychologists. The field is open for the evidence-based investigative psychology they practice. In fact, it has even been suggested that a new specialty, forensic media psychology, is on the horizon (Luskin, 2015).

Neuropsychology

Forensic psychologists are fascinated with deception detection. Several years ago, my first doctoral dissertation student wrote his dissertation on nonverbal body movement and deception. Every semester since, at least one student has decided to research another hypothesis regarding deception: blinking, micro expressions, foot movement, and other similar ideas. What nobody has tackled as yet, but what will most surely be a topic in the near future, is **functional magnetic resonance imaging (fMRI)**. The fMRI shows not only the state of the living brain, but also its processing actions. The development of fMRI and other neuroimaging technologies over the last three decades has enabled early diagnosis of brain lesions, led to claims that schizophrenia and other mental illness patterns and locations have been identified, and even provided new theories and confirmation of theories about areas of specific brain function (Fox, 2008; Perlin, 2009). One of the more recent theories is that since neuroimaging, particularly as manifested by the fMRI, has contributed so much to cognitive neuroscience, its ability to show function as well as state can be used to determine truth from lies and ultimately be used in courts for that purpose (Lucignani & Nappi, 2007). Companies using the fMRI commercially claim 90% accuracy in deception detection when this technology is used in employment and other nonlegal situations (Calderone, 2016).

If neuroimaging could actually provide this service, psychological study could have a profound impact on the legal system. As discussed elsewhere, existing lie detector "machines" simply record stress reactions, and there is no consensus that stress is equal to truth or deception (*Frye v. United States*, 1923). Further, some individuals do not seem to exhibit stress reactions. The fMRI actually reads brain activity, and some claim to understand what the readings mean (Calderone, 2016). One problem with the fMRI, however, is whether the theory can withstand critical scrutiny and earn admittance and acceptance into the legal system by way of the courts (Rusconi & Mitchener-Nissen, 2013). So far, no one has been able to replicate the claims of the one company that is apparently still in business (Calderone, 2016).[1] Issues raised regarding court use of this technology are admissibility of the results under the Federal Rules of Evidence (if the prejudicial effect would outweigh the probative value), the constitutionality of the evidence (the right against self-incrimination and due process rights), and the inability to replicate the accuracy claimed (Rusconi & Mitchener-Nissen, 2013). Other problems include violating a defendant's right to privacy and the fact that science is not absolutely sure what the fMRI is actually visualizing (Rusconi & Mitchener-Nissen, 2013). Meanwhile, technology has provided an exciting focus for forensic research and offers the potential for further expert psychological testimony.

Law Enforcement

The definition of forensic psychology seems to be constantly expanding as the need for psychologists in the legal system increases. This need includes law enforcement. Many students develop their interest in forensic psychology because of the media portrayals of forensic psychologists in such television shows as *Law and Order: Special Victims Unit* (Wolf, 1999–present) and *Criminal Minds* (Messer, 2005–present). In the former, several different actors have played forensic psychologists and psychiatrists over the 18 seasons the show has been running. Probably the most memorable role was that of Dr. George Huang, who was assigned to the Special Victims Unit. His character was so professional and respected in and by the fictional department that in 2004, the APA Division of Media Psychology presented the series with one of its highest honors (APA, 2004).[2] Just as Dr. Huang's role served a dual purpose on the show, so do forensic psychologists who work with law enforcement in real life. The psychologist may be there for the benefit of the police who require mental health services, to help evaluate police fitness for duty or recovery from traumatic situations, or in another capacity that might be of direct benefit to the department or its members (Kieliszewski, 2011).

Forensic psychologists may also be investigators for law enforcement. They may assess, strategize, negotiate, and perform psychological autopsies (see Chapter 6; Kieliszewski, 2011). Specifically, they may formulate a profile of a suspected perpetrator, as do the psychologists in *Criminal Minds* (Messer, 2005–present). The FBI does not call this type of prognostication profiling; it is "criminal investigative analysis" or **"investigative psychology"** (Winerman, 2004, para. 5). What *Criminal Minds* and the real FBI have in common, however, are their Behavioral Analysis Units (BAUs) (Halpern, 2011; Messer, 2005–present). The FBI's BAUs are made up of eight specially trained FBI agents, a crime analyst, and a major case specialist. Forensic psychologists are brought in from the military hospital outside the FBI (Halpern, 2011). The units also work with scientific and academic experts to amass as much information about a particular crime or crimes as possible (Marker, 2017). The BAU's goal is to find motivation for certain crimes; when they have accomplished that goal, they can usually find the perpetrator (Halpern, 2011). According to one BAU agent, the difference between the *Criminal Minds'* portrayal of the BAU and the actual one is that the BAU agents work with local law enforcement, investigate the crime or crimes, reach into their databases, and take a clinical, unemotional look at the evidence. They then give their findings to local law enforcement to use or not use as they see fit (Halpern, 2011).

Gangs

The study of gangs is an area of research for forensic psychology as well as a clinical problem for forensic psychologists working in law enforcement, correctional facilities, and the courts. Due to the proliferation of guns, drugs, and violent crime that gangs engender, police departments and other law enforcement agencies have special gang units dedicated to reducing gang violence, drug trafficking, and other gang-related crimes (see, for example, LAPD Gang and Narcotics Division and Chicago PD Gang Awareness). As will be seen in the "In the News" feature, street gangs are and have been a societal threat in most urban areas in the United States.

Theoretical research has not produced any solutions, but the more information psychology can amass regarding the reasons for gang membership and the violence that evolves from gang membership, the more weapons society in general and law enforcement in particular will have to curtail gang activities (Wood & Alleyne, 2010). Not only do gang members create fear and chaos on the streets, but they also are responsible for much prison violence and other misconduct, which in turn impacts forensic psychologists whose interest is in correctional psychology (Drury & DeLisi, 2011). Drury and DeLisi (2011) examined archival data of the prison population of one Southwestern state to determine the causes of misconduct by gang members in prison. Of the prisoners who were serving sentences for homicides of whatever degree, those who had or were suspected of having gang affiliations were also more likely to engage in prison misconduct. Their reasoning for this was that most homicides are crimes of passion, so those prisoners were for the most part single offenders. Gang members kill for notoriety and acceptance, and they carry that motivation into prison with them (Drury & DeLisi, 2011).

Correctional Psychology

As the prison population increases, the need for psychologists to work in prisons increases as well; in fact, inmates have three times the rate of mental illness as the general population (Benson, 2003). Prisons are building new units for mentally ill inmates and are providing internships as well as permanent positions for doctoral-level forensic psychologists (Davis, 2014; T. Elloyan, personal communication, March 2015). Research shows there is a need for mental health services in all correctional facilities, and when forensic psychology students get the opportunity to provide such services during their training years, they take full advantage of the experience.

Many of them stay on if offered positions to facilitate group therapy, plan programs, and counsel individuals when needed (see Dr. Trisha Elloyan interview, Chapter 4).[3]

Terrorism/Violence

While no discussion of the future of forensic psychology would be complete without mentioning terrorism and violence, so little is known about the motivation of individuals who commit those acts that prognosticating about the future of research is difficult at best (Horgan, 2017). Little is known about the mindset of the terrorist—or even if there is a mindset to be profiled (Johnson, 2016). However, from the psychological literature that is currently available, it seems obvious that if anyone is going to establish a profile of the would-be terrorist and assess risk at any given time in a given place, it would be a forensic psychologist.

The APA thought this topic was so important that it dedicated an entire issue of *American Psychologist* (2017) to it, with articles calling for research and risk assessment regarding potential terrorist activity. That particular journal issue could have been the result of previous controversy involving the APA and its involvement with "enhanced interrogation techniques" used by the Department of Defense (DoD) and the Central Intelligence Agency after the attacks on September 11, 2001, during the George W. Bush administration (Hoffman et al., 2015). In 2014, the APA hired a group of attorneys to conduct an independent investigation to determine if and to what extent APA member psychologists had ethically participated in government-conducted interrogations.

The report outlined a more than 10-year history of APA involvement with the DoD, "colluding with DoD officials to create and maintain loose APA ethics policies that did not significantly constrain DoD" interrogation methods (Hoffman et al., 2015, p. 9).[4] The findings in the report caused the APA to revise and rethink previous dealings with government departments and to finally pass a revision to its Standard 3.04 Avoiding Harm to include section (b), which explicitly states: "Psychologists do not participate in, facilitate, assist, or otherwise engage in torture, defined as any act by which severe pain or suffering, whether physical or mental, is intentionally inflicted on a person, or in any other cruel, inhuman, or degrading behavior that violates 3.04(a)" (APA, 2017c). While this revision leaves no doubt as to the APA's stand on torture, it comes too late for psychologists who were professionally involved with the government in advising on interrogation techniques and were apparently part of the "loose APA ethics policies" of the time. In August 2017, the Associated Press reported that a settlement had been reached between two psychologists "who helped design the CIA's harsh interrogation methods used in the war on terrorism" and clients of the American Civil Liberties Union who had been detainees of the United States (p. A22).

The Role of Diversity

Just as forensic psychology was implicitly involved in the issues related to the questionable ethics of some psychologists in regard to the "war on terror" in the United States, the role of diversity is implicitly part of every professional contact and decision made by the forensic psychologist (APA, 2013). Specialty Guidelines 2.07 and 2.08 caution forensic psychologists to consider the impact their personal beliefs and experiences may have on their ability to be impartial and the importance of appreciating individual and group differences.

Throughout these chapters, cases, articles, statutes, and the United States (U.S.) Constitution have been cited to implicitly or expressly show exactly what a diverse country we are. Courts have dealt with issues of racial, gender, and age discrimination as well as sexual preference, gender identity, mental health, and intellectual ability. Specialty Guideline 2.08 adds ethnicity, culture, national origin, religion, disability, language, and socioeconomic status to the list of differences that might need consideration (APA, 2013). Forensic psychologists need to know the boundaries of their impartiality and practice with competence. Guideline 2.07 admonishes that forensic practitioners may need to take steps to correct bias, decline participation if warranted, or limit their participation (APA, 2013). The caution is that we have legislated against discrimination but cannot legislate against prejudice, and the forensic psychologist needs to recognize that distinction.

SPOTLIGHT ON CASES

Death Penalty

Earlier chapters presented cases illustrating the U.S. Supreme Court's abolition of the death penalty for certain groups (*Atkins v. Virginia*, 2002; *Roper v. Simmons*, 2005). In those cases, some credit was given to the Amicus Curiae briefs of the APA for helping to persuade the Court to make those decisions. To date, the APA has filed 155 Amicus Curiae briefs; two of those briefs were filed in the cases that follow (Brief, 1984; Brief, 2017). As the future of forensic psychology is leading to a larger presence of these professionals in all facets of legal arenas, one very recent case illustrates the continuing influence the discipline has on the courts. The decision in *McWilliams v. Dunn* (2017) also illustrates the U.S. Supreme Court's reliance on precedent and desire for continuity.[5] First, the precedent-setting case follows.

Ake v. Oklahoma (1985)

Facts: Ake was charged with murdering a couple and wounding their children. While in custody, his behavior was so strange that the trial judge ordered a psychiatric evaluation and later a competency hearing. Ake was diagnosed with paranoid schizophrenia and determined to be incompetent to stand trial. Six weeks later, on medication, Ake was judged to be competent to stand trial. Defense counsel notified the court that Ake would be pleading insanity and asked for a full psychiatric evaluation at the state's expense, as Ake was indigent. The trial court rejected the argument, and although psychiatrists testified about Ake's mental condition at the time of examination, none could testify about his condition at the time of the offense. The U.S. Supreme Court noted that there was no expert testimony on either side regarding Ake's state of mind at the time of the offense. He was found guilty. During sentencing, he again had no expert testifying, but the court relied on the state's psychiatrist, who said he presented a danger to society, and sentenced him to death.

Procedural History: The Oklahoma appeals court agreed with the lower court that the Constitution did not require the state to provide psychiatric services to indigent defendants. The U.S. Supreme Court granted certiorari.

Issue: Does the U.S. Constitution require the state to provide psychiatric/psychological services to an indigent defendant?

Rule/Holding: All defendants are entitled to all the assistance necessary for an effective defense. When mental health is raised as an issue, the defendant is entitled to the services of a competent mental health expert who can evaluate, assist, and present the case to the trier of fact. The facts of this case make clear that this defendant could have a fair trial and sentencing only if the mental health factors he raised were taken into consideration.

Judgment: Reversed and remanded.

And 32 years later:

McWilliams v. Dunn (2017)

Facts: James McWilliams was charged with rape and murder in Alabama 1 month after the Supreme Court's decision in *Ake v. Oklahoma*. McWilliams was found to be indigent and was provided with counsel, who moved for a pretrial psychiatric evaluation. Three psychiatrists examined the defendant and agreed he was competent to stand trial and that he was not suffering from mental illness at the time of the rape and murder. The defense counsel was hoping to mitigate the sentence. The testimony of the psychiatrists gave the impression they felt McWilliams was malingering and exaggerating his symptoms. He was convicted. During his sentencing hearing, McWilliams and his mother testified that he had suffered brain injuries as a child and had a series of psychiatric and psychological evaluations. One psychological evaluation diagnosed a psychotic thought disorder with need for inpatient treatment. The jury recommended the death sentence; Alabama law required that 10 of 12 jurors agree to a sentence, and 10 agreed that McWilliams be sentenced to death. Although two psychologists spent sufficient time evaluating McWilliams, their evaluations and other mental health records did not reach the defense in time for counsel to read, understand, and present them at the sentencing hearing. The judge denied all defense motions for continuation, stated he had reviewed the records, and decided McWilliams was faking; even if he was not faking, the judge said, there were enough aggravating factors in the case to impose the death sentence.

Procedural History: McWilliams appealed the sentence to the state appeals court which affirmed the sentence, stating that McWilliams had an opportunity to call a psychologist to testify for him but did not—the opportunity was all the *Ake* decision required. The Alabama Supreme Court affirmed the decision. McWilliams appealed to federal court, claiming he was denied the constitutional rights that *Ake* required. The federal courts affirmed the state decisions, and McWilliams appealed to the U.S. Supreme Court.

Background: The appeal to the U.S. Supreme Court was based on its ruling in *Ake*, which stated that three conditions had to be met for *Ake* to be applied: (1) an indigent defendant, (2) whose mental condition is relevant to the punishment, and (3) whose mental condition was seriously in question at the time of the offense.

Issue: Did the record show that McWilliams received the mental health expertise required by the *Ake* decision?

Holding: *Ake* requires that the defendant receive mental health expertise for examination, to assist in evaluation, preparation, and presentation of the defense. The facts here show that the only part of the *Ake* requirements McWilliams received was the examination.

Judgment: Reversed for petitioner and remanded.

Although the *McWilliams* case clearly depended on the precedent set in the *Ake* case, it is interesting to note that *Ake v. Oklahoma* had only one dissenting opinion in 1985. *McWilliams v. Dunn* was a much closer 5–4 decision in 2017. Even more important is that McWilliams was sentenced 31 years before this case finally went to the U.S. Supreme Court.

IN THE NEWS

As has been seen throughout this book, any one of the forensic psychology topics could be a news story on any given day. In fact, while reading a daily newspaper or watching the news on one device or another, it becomes habit to think about the role the forensic psychologist might play in almost any domestic violence, violence, terrorism, or school shooting report. Veterans' rights, prison and jail issues, prisoner exonerations, police misconduct, and juvenile delinquency are all subjects for the expertise of a forensic psychologist. Those, of course, are only the topics that make the news; child custody, disability, and probate matters rarely make the news, but are certainly no less important to the individuals dealing with the problems. However, in a chapter emphasizing the growth of forensic psychology and its future, elaborating on two subjects raised in the chapter is appropriate.

MS-13 Gang

In May 2017, the Los Angeles Chief of Police, Charlie Beck, announced that his department, with the cooperation of several federal agencies, raided multiple premises and arrested over 20 members of the MS-13 gang. The arrests came as a result of a 2-year investigation into the crimes of the violent gang. Twenty people had already been arrested, and the police were looking for three more. The acting U.S. Attorney said the arrests should put a large hole in the MS-13 leadership. Although many of the gang members who were arrested were in the country illegally, MS-13 is known to prey on other undocumented individuals through extortion, robbery, rape, and murder. The police chief acknowledged that without the cooperation of these innocent undocumented workers, law enforcement never could have collected enough evidence against the gang members to arrest and charge them (Winton, 2017).

Brain Damage and Criminal Defense

Relevant to both the topic of neuropsychology and the case of James McWilliams is the defense of brain damage asserted by Andres "Andy" Avalos, who was charged with murdering his wife, a neighbor, and a pastor (Davis, 2017). The defense claimed that a brain scan showed he had a "severely abnormal brain" (Davis, 2017, p. A11). Kevin Davis (2017), who wrote the article, mentioned several other murderers who claimed brain damage made them do it. He also wrote a book called *The Brain Defense: Murder in Manhattan and the Dawn of Neuroscience* (2017). The brain damage defense, according to Davis, is appropriate and responsibly used if it goes to sentencing. For those pleading a mental defect, as was seen in earlier chapters, the burden is on the defendant to show that but for the brain injury, the crime would not have occurred.

Davis wrote the article for the *Los Angeles Times* on May 3, 2017. On May 22, 2017, Avalos was sentenced to life in prison (WFLA Web Staff, 2017). The prosecution had been requesting the death penalty.

SUMMARY

This final chapter addressed the future of forensic psychology and its growth. To do that, new topics were introduced to show the breadth of the discipline. First, forensic psychology and its relationship to the APA were explored. The APA has well over 100,000 members, and its influence and the opportunities the organization makes available are international in scope (APA history, 2017b). Media psychology, neuropsychology, police, gangs, correctional psychology, and terrorism/violence are all potential areas of specialized practice for forensic psychologists. Forensic psychologists are informally guided by the *Specialty Guidelines for Forensic Psychology* (2013). Examining two of them in regard to the importance of diversity considerations was also part of the chapter. Finally, two cases specifically related to the work of mental health experts were briefed. These cases illustrated the need for mental health experts, issues raised by death penalty sentencing, and the importance of consistency and precedent in the U.S. Supreme Court.

DISCUSSION QUESTIONS

1. There are many types of forensic careers beside psychology. Discuss some of them and explain how the practitioners' expertise might be utilized.
2. Discuss some other constitutional and/or legal issues that admitting fMRI results into criminal prosecutions might raise.

Do you think criminal defendants claiming innocence could someday be required to submit to an fMRI? What issues might that requirement raise?

3. What is your understanding of the differences in the APA's Principles, Standards, and Specialty Guidelines for Forensic Psychologists?

4. James McWilliams had been on "death row" for 31 years when the U.S. Supreme Court decided his case in 2017. Discuss your thoughts about the death penalty, both as a sentence and in its application.

NOTES

1. As of July 2017, No Lie MRI's website was at http://www.noliemri.com/centers/Overview.htm.

2. The Division of Media Psychology is now Division 46, Society for Media Psychology and Technology.

3. Dr. Elloyan is one of three of my former students who recently were offered positions in prisons. Two of them are in California, and one is in North Carolina.

4. The entire report is available at https://www.apa.org/independent-review/APA-FINAL-Report-7.2.15.pdf.

5. The interest in continuity of the U.S. Supreme Court is even more notable with these two cases. Not one of the justices on the Court for the *Ake v. Oklahoma* decision was still on the court for the *McWilliams v. Dunn* decision.

REFERENCES

Ake v. Oklahoma, 470 U.S. 68 (1985). Retrieved from http://www.apa.org/about/apa/archives/apa-history.aspx

American Psychologist. (2017, April). American Psychological Association. Retrieved from http://psycnet.apa.org/fulltext/2017-13879-001.pdf

American Psychological Association. (APA). (2004). APA gives awards to television's *Law & Order: Special Victims Unit* and journalist Patricia Bellinghausen. Retrieved from http://www.apa.org/news/press/releases/2004/07/media-awards.aspx

American Psychological Association. (APA). (2013). Specialty guidelines for forensic psychology. *American Psychologist, 68*(1), 7–19. doi:10.1037/a0029889.

American Psychological Association. (APA). (2017a). *APA accredited.* Search for accredited programs. Retrieved from http://apps.apa.org/accredsearch/?_ga=2.112732995.694279839.1502776251-1567043931.1482877825

American Psychological Association. (APA). (2017b). *APA history.* Retrieved from http://www.apa.org/about/apa/archives/apa-history.aspx

American Psychological Association. (APA). (2017c). *Ethical principles of psychologists and code of conduct.* Washington, DC: Author. Retrieved from http://www.apa.org/ethics/code/ethics-code-2017.pdf.

Associated Press. (2017, August 20). Legal settlement in psychologists' CIA torture case. *Los Angeles Times*, p. A 22.

Benson, E. (2003). Rehabilitate or punish? *Monitor, 34*(7), 46.

Brief for the American Psychological Association as Amicus Curiae in support of petitioner, footnote, *Ake v. Oklahoma* 470 U.S. 68 (1985).

Brief for the American Psychological Association as Amicus Curiae in support of petitioner, *McWilliams v. Dunn*, No. 165294 (2017).

Bureau of Labor Statistics. (2016). *National occupational employment and wage estimates.* Retrieved from https://www.bls.gov/oes/current/oes193039.htm

Calderone, J. (2016). There are some big problems with brain scan lie detectors. *Business Insider.* Retrieved from http://www.businessinsider.com/dr-oz-huizenga-fmri-brain-lie-detector-2016-4

CAPIC. (2017). *CAPIC takes steps to reduce the national psychology internship crisis.* Retrieved from http://capic.net/wp-content/uploads/2014/08/CAPIC-Outreach-to-Out-of-State-Doctoral-Programs-updated-gw.pdf

Davis, K. (2014, January 2). New prison unit for disabled, mentally ill. *San Diego Union-Tribune.* Retrieved from http://www.sandiegouniontribune.com/sdut-donovan-new-prison-unit-disabled-mentally-ill-2014jan02-story.html

Davis, K. (2017, May 3). Why are lawyers using brain damage as a criminal defense? The science doesn't support it. *Los Angeles Times*, A11.

Drury, A. J., & DeLisi, M. (2011). Gangkill: An exploratory empirical assessment of gang membership, homicide offending, and prison misconduct. *Crime & Delinquency, 57*(1), 130–146.

Fox, D. (2008). Brain imaging and the Bill of Rights: Memory detection technologies and American criminal justice. *American Journal of Bioethics, 8*(1), 34–36. doi:10.1080/15265160701828451

Halpern, M. (host). (2011, May 2). *Behavior analysts: Making sense of the incomprehensible. Inside the FBI* [Audio podcast]. Retrieved from https://www.fbi.gov/audio-repository/news-podcasts-inside-bau-profilers.mp3/view

Hoffman, D. H., Carter, D .J., Lopez, C. R. V., Benzmiller, H. L., Guo, A. X., Latifi, S. Y., & Craig, D. C. (2015). Report to the special committee of the board of directors of the American Psychological Association: Independent review relating to APA ethics guidelines, national security interrogations, and torture. Retrieved from https://www.apa.org/independent-review/APA-FINAL-Report-7.2.15.pdf

Hoffman v. State No.540.2011 (2012).

Horgan, J. G. (2017). Psychology of terrorism: Introduction to the special issue. *American Psychologist, 72*(3), 199–204. Retrieved from http://dx.doi.org/10.1037/amp0000148

Jenkins v. United States 307 F.2d 637 (D.C. Cir.1962).

Johnson, R. (2016). Forensic psychological mindset of a terrorist: More questions than answers for public safety threat risk assessments. *Security Journal, 29*(2), 185–197.

Kieliszewski, J. (2011). Forensic psychology and law enforcement: Police and investigative psychology. *Current Perspectives in Criminal Psychology.* Retrieved from http://criminalpsychologytoday.blogspot.com/2011/04/forensic-psychology-and-law-enforcement.html

Lucignani, G., & Nappi, G. (2007). Neuroimaging technology and philosophy: A coming of age. *Functional Neurology, 22*(4), 181–183.

Luskin, B. J. (2015). Forensic media psychology and a camera in every pocket. *Psychology Today.* Retrieved from https://www.psychologytoday.com/blog/the-media-psychology-effect/201504/forensic-media-psychology-and-camera-in-every-pocket

Marker, V. (2017). Forensic psychology: A less traveled law enforcement career path. *PoliceOne.* Retrieved from https://www.policeone.com/police-jobs-and-careers/articles/3702021-Forensic-psychology-A-less-traveled-law-enforcement-career-path/

McWilliams v. Dunn, No. 16-5294 (2017)

Messer, E. (Producer) (2005–present). *Criminal Minds* [Television series]. The Mark Gordon Company in association with CBS Television Studios and ABC Studios.

People v. Spriggs, Fo66927 (2014).

Perlin, M. L. (2009). "His brain has been mismanaged with great skill": How will jurors respond to neuroimaging testimony in insanity defense cases? *Akron Law Review, 42*, 885–916.

Rusconi, E., & Mitchener-Nissen, T. (2013). Prospects of functional magnetic resonance imaging as lie detector. *Frontiers in Human Neuroscience, 7*, Article 594, 1–12.

United States v. Anderson, No. 11-2121(8th Cir. 2012).

WFLA Web Staff. (2017, May 22). Life in prison for Avalos. *News Channel 8: On your side*. Retrieved from http://wfla.com/2017/05/22/andres-avalos-sentenced-to-life/

White v. White, Superior Court of New Jersey, Chancery Division, Union County (2001).

Winerman, L. (2004). Criminal profiling: The reality behind the myth. *Monitor*. Retrieved from http://www.apa.org/monitor/julaug04/criminal.aspx

Winton, R. (2017, May 17). Early morning raids end in arrests of nearly two dozen MS-13 gang suspects. *Los Angeles Times*. Retrieved from http://www.latimes.com/local/lanow/la-me-ln-ms13-sweep-20170517-story.html

Wolf, D. (Producer). (1999–present). *Law and Order: SVU* [Television series]. Wolf Films in association with Universal Television.

Wood, J., & Alleyne, E. (2010). Street gang theory and research: Where are we now and where do we go from here? *Aggression and Violent Behavior*, 15(2), 100–111.

INDEX